SHOULDER PAIN

EDITION 2

SHOULDER PAIN

RENE CAILLIET, M.D.

Professor and Chairman
Department of Rehabilitative Medicine
University of Southern California
School of Medicine
Los Angeles, California

 F. A. DAVIS COMPANY • Philadelphia

Also by Rene Cailliet:

FOOT AND ANKLE PAIN
HAND PAIN AND IMPAIRMENT
KNEE PAIN AND DISABILITY
LOW BACK PAIN SYNDROME
NECK AND ARM PAIN
SCOLIOSIS
SOFT TISSUE PAIN AND DISABILITY
THE SHOULDER IN HEMIPLEGIA

Printed in the United States of America

**Library of Congress Cataloging in Publication
Data**

Cailliet, René.
    Shoulder pain.

    Bibliography: p.
    Includes index.
    1. Shoulder—Diseases. 2. Pain. I. Title.
[DNLM: 1. Pain—Therapy. 2. Shoulder
WE 810 C134s]
RC939.C36 1981   617′.572   80-27750
ISBN 0-8036-1613-9

Preface

Pain in the shoulder region is exceeded in clinical frequency only by pain in the low back and pain in the neck. Recent developments and modifications of older concepts concerning shoulder pain, together with the need for further clarification of associated disease syndromes, have prompted this new edition.

The shoulder remains a complex functional unit with numerous tissues capable of causing joint dysfunction. As in all musculoskeletal systems, a thorough knowledge of functional anatomy is mandatory, and the examiner must evaluate every aspect of this functional anatomy. Treatment must, therefore, be based on modification or correction of these malfunctions. The shoulder joints, some eight or nine in number, may all contribute to pain and dysfunction, thus methodical examination, individually and collectively, of all these joints must be performed.

When man began to assume the upright position, and his forelegs became arms and hands, the shoulder and its arm components became useful to place the hand in functional position and to acquire greater mobility at the expense of stability. Due to this lack of stability, degeneration, damage, pain, and malfunction can result.

This new edition is meant to supplement the previous one. Its organization is basically the same in that functional anatomy is stressed, and examination to determine any deviation from normal can be appreciated. The patient's history and examination thus become meaningful, and treatment evolves from this concept, based on physiologic principles.

New chapters have been added which involve the hemiplegic shoulder and the shoulder-hand-finger syndrome, both of which are seen constantly in daily practice. The bibliography has been chosen to update current references to the concepts postulated.

RENE CAILLIET, M.D.

Contents

Illustrations

ix

Introduction

The complaint of pain in the upper extremity can present a confusing diagnostic problem to the practitioner and to the therapist. The upper extremity includes the anterior and posterior angles of the neck, shoulder, arm, elbow, wrist, and hand. Pain can originate from these tissues or may be felt in these tissues as a referred pain from other areas.

The outline appearing on pages 40 and 41 enumerates the major causes of pain in the upper extremity. Obviously, exhaustive consideration of all these causes is not possible in a single monograph. Since the predominant causes seen in daily clinical practice belong in the musculoskeletal system, these will be stressed.

Degenerative causes affecting the shoulder girdle and its numerous joints cannot be completely differentiated from other causes of inflammation or from trauma.

This examination is grounded in biomechanical physiology, which classifies the glenohumeral joint as an incongruous joint. The congruity which affords stability to a joint and limited motion also must be studied in conjunction with incongruity, such as that of the glenohumeral joint, which permits excessive mobility and inadequate stability, thus providing the basis for pain, degeneration, and dysfunction.

Terminology used in reference to the upper extremity, especially with regard to the shoulder girdle, is vague, nonspecific, and arbitrary. Many hackneyed terms have gained dignity of specificity but are loosely employed, devoid of real meaning, and without physiologic basis. As their use becomes well established, these meaningless terms, invoking no pathomechanical concept, are bound to lead to inadequate treatment and persistence of pain and disability. This text is intended to furnish a sound functional pathophysiologic basis for understanding pain and dysfunction of the shoulder.

The purpose of this new edition is to provide the clinician with a sound basis for performing a significant history and a meaningful examination, and for prescribing rational treatment for the patient who complains of pain in the shoulder region, in the upper extremity as related to the shoulder, or in the shoulder emanating from other portions of the musculoskeletal system. Hopefully, better prescription for treatment and better functional evaluations will result, and the physical and occupational therapists who are assigned the responsibility of providing treatment will have recourse to clearer and more reliable guidelines.

CHAPTER 1

Functional Anatomy

The term *shoulder joint* requires elucidation. The common use of the term *joint*, referring to the glenohumeral joint, refers to only one of the seven joints that form the shoulder complex. Since all the joints comprising the complex are separately and collectively important in normal function, and since impairment of one may cause impairment of all, a collective term is desirable. The term *shoulder girdle* is preferable if it enjoys the definition of "arm-trunk mechanism," "thoracic-scapular-humeral articulation," or "shoulder-arm complex."

The shoulder girdle is a composite of seven joints all moving synchronously, each incumbent upon the other, with dysfunction resulting from the impairment of any of the participating joints. Rhythmic movement of the arm upon the chest wall is totally dependent for its *mobility* upon coordinated muscular action and for its *stability* upon combined muscular and ligamentous structures.

When man became an erect individual, his arms, which in his quadriped state were his forelegs, gave up anatomical and functional stability in favor of mobility. Consequently the shoulder girdle in man has sacrificed stability for mobility which is the greatest of all the joints of the body.

Analysis of total movement of the shoulder girdle proceeds best if each joint is considered separately, rather than the total combined. Admittedly, this separate approach is unphysiologic because the shoulder complex functions by synchronous movements occurring simultaneously in a smooth, integrated manner, which is aptly described as the "scapulohumeral rhythm" by Dr. E. A. Codman.[1] The individual joint approach permits simplicity of inspection and evaluation and facilitates ultimate integration into the complex.

The component joints of the shoulder girdle are shown in Figure 1. These joints can be enumerated in reverse order from the legend of Figure 1, beginning with the first and only attachment to the vertebral

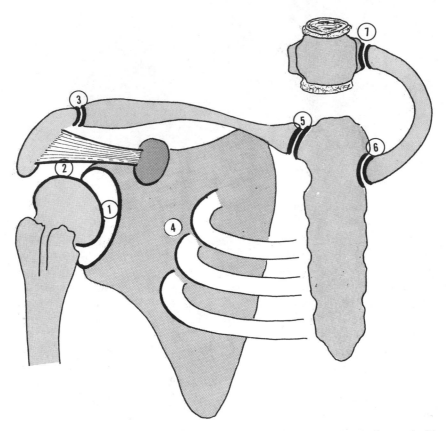

FIGURE 1. The joints of the shoulder girdle: (1) glenohumeral; (2) suprahumeral; (3) acromioclavicular; (4) scapulocostal; (5) sternoclavicular; (6) costosternal; (7) costovertebral.

column. All other contiguous joints are extrinsic to the vertebral column.

The initial joint is the joint between the ribs and the vertebral body, the *costovertebral joint*. The next contiguous joint is the *costosternal joint*, followed by the *sternoclavicular joint*. The remaining articulation of the trunk portion of the girdle is the *scapulocostal joint*. The first three joints mentioned conform more to the accepted definition of a joint in that they are unions of two bones that permit movement at their junction.[2] The scapulocostal joint conforms only equivocally to the definition: it is a gliding joint of the scapula with the rib cage separated by muscles and a bursa.

The arm portion of the arm-trunk complex, at best an arbitrary division, begins with the *acromioclavicular joint*. The sixth joint is the *suprahumeral joint*, which is also a functional joint rather than a true

2

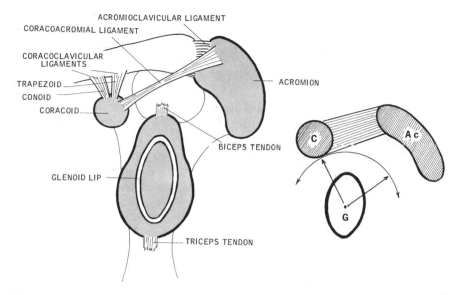

FIGURE 2. The acromiocoracoid arch. The diagram depicts the shape of the glenoid fossa and its relationship to the acromial process, the coracoid process, and the coracoacromial ligament. In essence this diagram shows the socket of the glenohumeral joint and also portrays the relationship of the suprahumeral joint.

joint. This "joint" refers to the relationship of the humeral head to the overlying coracoacromial arch (Fig. 2). Although alluded to as a "pseudo" joint, the relationship of this joint is extremely important in the normal movement of the shoulder girdle and is an integral part in many of the pathologic states.

The seventh joint commonly considered *the* shoulder joint is the *glenohumeral joint*. An additional articulation that has pathologic significance but little functional importance is the *biceps mechanism*, a gliding articulation of the biceps tendon within the bicipital groove. Actually, the tendon does *not* glide within the groove, but stays fixed, and the humerus glides along the tendon. This gliding motion occurs during any and all movement of the shoulder joint. Flexing and spinating the forearm upon the humerus, a biceps action, causes the biceps tendon to become taut but not to glide or move within the bicipital groove.

Each of the enumerated joints will be considered separately, then the coordinated motion involving all these single actions will be analyzed. Failure of any component movement will cause failure of the composite movement of the shoulder girdle. The clinical examination inspects each movement as well as the complex movement. Examination also reveals the defect in the mechanism that, coupled with the history, gives a mechanical diagnosis and a rational treatment aimed at restoring normal function to the impaired component and restitution of the "scapulohumeral rhythm."

GLENOHUMERAL JOINTS

The *glenohumeral joint,* part 1 in Figure 1, may be termed the scapulohumeral joint and the joint that is most commonly termed *the shoulder joint.*

The glenohumeral joint is a classic example of an *incongruous* joint. In a *congruous* joint the surfaces are symmetrical or parallel with the concave surface, and the convex opposing surfaces are equidistant (Fig. 3A). The convex surface is roundly cylindrical, whereas the incongruous joint's surfaces are oval.

In the congruous joints, rotation occurs about a fixed central axis. Rotation of the inserting joint's surface occurs about this stationary axis, and thus the muscles that move it have equal action upon the moving part. This congruous joint relationship affords stability insofar as the ball-socket relationship *seats* the head within the socket. The capsule, also about a symmetrical joint, extends equally in all directions during movement.

The incongruous joint, having a shallow concave surface that articulates with a more convex and thus dissimilar surface, loses its relationship. The incongruous joint is thus not in a ball-socket relationship and is unstable. The convex portion of the joint does not seat itself into the shallow concave portion (Fig. 3B).

Movement of the incongruous joint is not rotation about a fixed axis, but rather a gliding motion about a constantly changing axis of rotation. The muscles thus must not only move the joint, but must also afford it its stability. The capsule of an incongruous joint must have greater flexibility as it is extended further during the gliding activity.

The *glenohumeral joint* is an example of an incongruous joint with all the factors of this type of joint affecting normal movement and contributing to pain and disability.

The scapula, the "shoulder blade" (Fig. 4), lies on the posterior surface of the thoracic cage with its ventral surface concave, corresponding to the convex surface of the rib cage. The only attachments to the thorax and spinal column other than the acromioclavicular joint are muscular.

The dorsal surface of the scapula is divided by the *spine,* a horizontal bony ridge that extends laterally past the glenoid fossa ending in a bulbous end, the *acromial process.* This process overhangs the head of the humerus, is the site of attachment to the clavicle (the acromioclavicular joint), and receives the fibers of the coracoacromial liga-

4

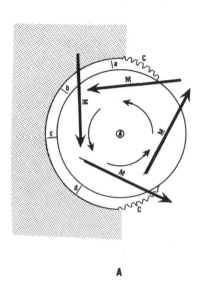
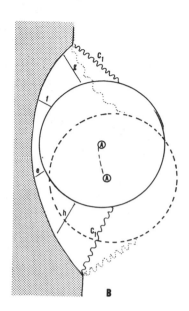

A   B

FIGURE 3. Congruous-incongruous joints. *A*. In a congruous joint the concave, convex surfaces are symmetrical. The articular surfaces are equidistant from each other at all points along their circumference (a = b = c = d, etc.). In rotation, movement occurs about a fixed axis (A). Muscular action (M) is that of symmetrical movement about this fixed axis and is needed for motion, not stability. The depth of the concave surface gives the joint stability. The capsule (C) has symmetrical elongation. *B*. Incongruous joints have asymmetrical articulatory surfaces. The concave surface is elongated and the convex more circular, thus the distance between them varies at each point (g > f > e < h). As the joint moves, the axis of rotation (A) shifts and joint movement is that of gliding rather than rolling. Therefore, muscles must slide the joint and simultaneously maintain stability. The capsule varies in its elongation at all levels of movement. The glenohumeral joint is an incongruous joint.

ment. The acromion and the coracoacromial ligament form part of the arch overlying the suprahumeral joint (see Fig. 2).

The glenoid fossa, the female portion of the glenohumeral joint, is located on the anterior superior angle of the scapula, midway between and below the acromion and the coracoid process. The glenoid fossa is a shallow, ovoid socket that faces anteriorly, laterally, and upward (Fig. 4). The direction upward has clinical significance in furnishing stability to the glenohumeral joint.

Surrounding the perimeter of the fossa, to deepen the cup, is a fibrous lip known as the *glenoid labrum*. This lip, originally considered to be fibrocartilage,[2] contains no cartilage but is primarily fibrous tissue, a redundant fold of the anterior capsule.[3] This fold, and apparently the labrum, disappears as the humerus is externally rotated.

There is marked discrepancy between the surface area and the

5

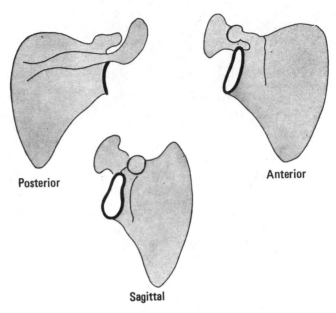

Posterior

Anterior

Sagittal

FIGURE 4. The scapula. The posterior, anterior, and sagittal views of the scapula are shown. The spine of the scapula seen on the posterior view divides the blade into the supra- and infraspinatus fossae, from which originate the muscles that also bear these names. The sagittal view is more graphically seen in Figure 2, which depicts the relationship of the glenoid fossa to the overhanging acromial process and the medially located coracoid process. Note the angle of the glenoid fossa, facing laterally, anteriorly, and upward.

curvature of the glenoid fossa and the convex surface of the humeral head. Only a small portion of the head of the humerus is in contact with the fossa at any time. This incongruous joint relationship demands a gliding joint movement rather than the ball-bearing type of joint in the hip. This unstable but mobile relationship requires synchronous muscular actions for its movements.

GLENOHUMERAL CAPSULE

The capsule of the glenohumeral joint is an extremely thin-walled, spacious container that attaches around the entire perimeter of the glenoid rim. A small portion of the epiphyseal line of the glenoid extends within the capsule, which is the reason that osteomyelitis can sometimes extend into the articular space.

As shown in Figure 5, the capsule arises from the glenoid fossa and inserts around the anatomical neck of the humerus. There is a synovial lining throughout that blends with the hyaline cartilage of the

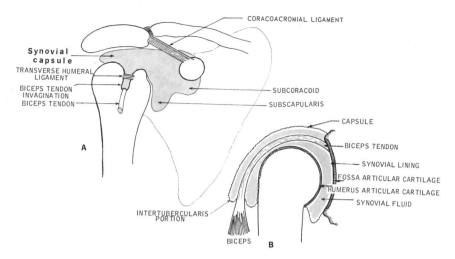

FIGURE 5. The glenohumeral synovial capsule. *A*. The spacious capsule covers the entire humeral head. The invagination of the capsule accompanying the biceps tendon down the bicipital groove passes under the transverse humeral ligament at the level of the point of attachment of the pectoralis major muscle to the shaft of the humerus. The subscapularis and subcoracoid pouches of the capsule contain synovial fluid and are in direct continuity with the major capsule. These pouches are clearly seen in dye arthrograms. *B*. The intracapsular, extrasynovial invagination of the long head of the biceps tendon as it proceeds to attach to the superior rim of the glenoid fossa. The synovial lining attaches to the articular cartilage of the head of the humerus but attaches to the glenoid fossa at a distance from the rim of the glenoid cartilage.

head of the humerus but fails to reach the cartilage of the glenoid fossa (Fig. 5*B*).

The long head of the biceps attaches to the superior aspect of the glenoid fossa (see Fig. 2). It invaginates the capsule but *does not enter the synovial cavity*. The biceps tendon is thus *intracapsular* but remains *extrasynovial*. The capsule folds and incorporates the biceps tendon down into the intertubercular sulcus of the humerus and ends blindly at a site on the humerus opposite the insertion of the pectoralis major muscle (Fig. 5*A*).[4]

With the arm hanging loosely in a dependent position at the side, the upper portion of the capsule is taut, and the inferior portion, the axillary fold, is loose and pleated (Fig. 6). The opposite situation exists when the arm is fully *abducted*. Here the inferior portion becomes taut and the superior portion pleated. The tautness of the superior capsule with the arm dependent prevents downward dislocation of the arm, and the laxity of the capsule permits the gliding motion of the glenohumeral joint.

Rotation of the arm around its longitudinal axis (turning the arm in

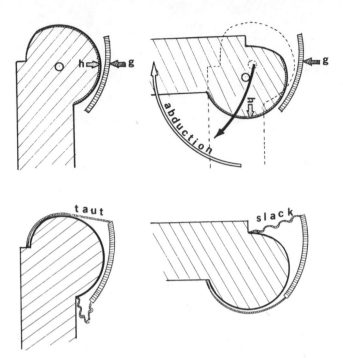

FIGURE 6. Capsular action during glenohumeral movement. The upper drawing depicts the "gliding" joint motion between the head of the humerus and the glenoid fossa. The arc of both joint surfaces differ and thus form an incongruous joint surface relationship. The lower left drawing shows the arm dependent with the superior portion of the capsule taut, which prevents downward movement. The lower right drawing shows the arm abducted, which relaxes the superior portion of the capsule and causes the inferior portion to become taut. In the half-abducted arm both superior and inferior capsules are slack, which position is thus one of instability of the glenohumeral joint.

and out and to and from the trunk, while dependent) has the same effect of tautness and laxity upon the capsule, anteriorly and posteriorly. The anterior portion of the capsule is reinforced by the superior, middle, and inferior *glenohumeral ligaments*. These ligaments are actually pleated horizontal *folds* of the anterior capsule in a fan-shaped appearance in front of the glenohumeral joint. These fan-shaped ligaments have a base attached on the humerus and converge toward the glenoid rim, some distance in from the edge of the fossa, to attach on the anterior superior portion of the glenoid and the adjacent bone (Fig. 7).

There is a recess, a pouch, in the anterior capsule due to the looseness of the capsule. The capsule is actually loose enough to permit the humerus to be drawn as much as 3 cm from the fossa. An opening usually exists between the superior and middle glenohumeral ligaments (folds), termed the foramen of Weitbrecht, which is merely

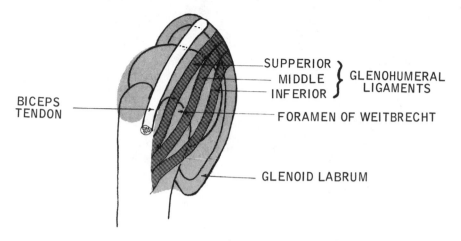

BICEPS
TENDON

SUPPERIOR ⎫
MIDDLE ⎬ GLENOHUMERAL
INFERIOR ⎭ LIGAMENTS

FORAMEN OF WEITBRECHT

GLENOID LABRUM

FIGURE 7. The anterior capsule and the glenohumeral ligaments. The glenohumeral ligaments that reinforce the anterior joint capsule are mere folds of the capsule. Three in number, they are fan-shaped, attach from the humerus, and converge toward the glenoid rim. The foramen of Weitbrecht may be covered by a thin layer or may be open as a communication between the joint space and the subscapular recess.

covered by a thin layer of capsule, or may be open as a communication between the joint capsule and the subscapular recess. The anterior pouch, due to capsular laxity and the foramen of Weitbrecht, assumes significance in dislocations of the humerus.[5]

Limitation of external rotation upon the glenoid fossa is also imposed by the coracohumeral ligament (Fig. 8). This ligament originates at the coracoid process of the scapula and attaches to the humerus at the bicipital groove upon the bone and the ligament of the biceps tendon. In active or passive external rotation of the humerus this ligament acts to limit the extent of rotation. Constriction of this ligament is considered to play a role in the "frozen shoulder," or limited adhesive capsulitis.

THE SUPRAHUMERAL JOINT

The *suprahumeral joint* is not a joint in the true sense: an articulation, more or less moveable, between two or more bones.[6] The suprahumeral joint is more a protective articulation between the head of the humerus and an arch formed by a broad, triangular ligament connecting the acromial process and the coracoid process (see Fig. 2).

The coracoacromial arch prevents trauma from above to the glenohumeral joint or to the head of the humerus and also prevents upward dislocation of the humerus. Its proximity to the humerus in its inner aspect presents an obstacle to abduction of the humerus in the

9

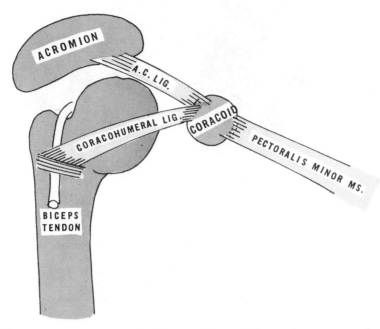

FIGURE 8. The coracohumeral ligament.

coronal plane (see Fig. 15). This will be discussed in the section on composite shoulder girdle movements.

The suprahumeral articulation is bounded within by the glenoid cavity, superiorly and slightly posteriorly by the acromial process, anteriorly and medially by the coracoid process, and above by the coracoacromial ligament. The humeral head lies under this hood.

Within the suprahumeral joint are found portions of the subacromial bursa, the subcoracoid bursa, the supraspinatus muscle and its tendon, the superior portion of the glenohumeral capsule, a portion of the biceps tendon, and the interposed loose connective tissue. Many sensitive tissues are enclosed within this small area.[7,8]

As the arm abducts, the greater tuberosity must pass under the coracoacromial ligament and not compress the enclosed tissues. The movement requires fine muscular coordination, laxity of soft tissues, and proper external rotation of the humerus. Impairment of any of these factors can result in limited movement, pain, and disability.

MUSCULATURE OF THE GLENOHUMERAL JOINT

Five of the nine muscles related to the glenohumeral joint can be considered the prime movers. The more complex in their movement are those collectively known as the *musculotendinous cuff muscles*.

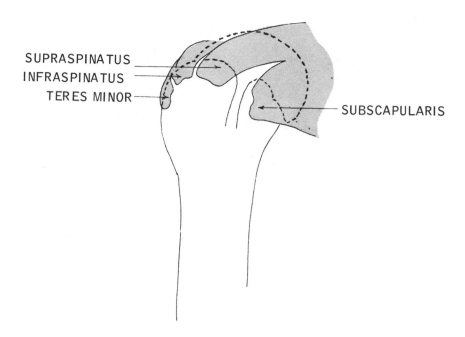

SUPRASPINATUS
INFRASPINATUS
TERES MINOR

SUBSCAPULARIS

FIGURE 9. Rotator cuff insertion upon the humerus. The conjoined tendinous insertion of the four rotator muscles that comprise the "cuff" is viewed anteriorly. The supraspinatus attaches to the greater tuberosity; the infraspinatus, immediately below it; and then the teres minor. The subscapularis inserts upon the lesser tuberosity below the cartilage of the head and medial to the bicipital groove. There is a sulcus through which the biceps tendon emerges.

The important motions of the glenohumeral joint are performed by these cuff muscles. Through their attachment to the humerus they act as rotators and combine with the deltoid muscle to abduct the arm by producing various combinations of force couples about the glenohumeral joint (Fig. 9).

The cuff muscles, especially the supraspinatus muscle, passively support the dependent humerus in the person standing or sitting. The arm at the glenohumeral articulation would dislocate downward out of the socket if it were not for the cuff support and the angle of the glenoid fossa (Fig. 10).

The *rotator* action of the cuff muscles relates to rotation around a point located in the center of the head of the humerus in an arc of the sagittal plane. This rotation differs from rotation around the long shaft of the humerus, as in internal and external rotation of the arm.

The muscles comprising the *rotator cuff* are the supraspinatus, infraspinatus, teres minor, and the subscapularis muscles.

The *supraspinatus muscle* originates from the supraspinatus fossa

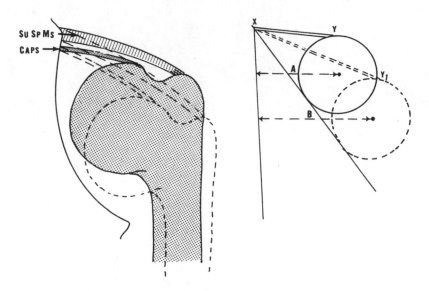

FIGURE 10. Capsular-passive cuff support. Due to the orientation of the glenoid fossa which faces forward, outward, and upward, the superior capsule, being taut in the normal position, becomes more taut as the humeral head (A) descends. B depicts an analogy of a ball rolling down an angled plane.

of the scapula above the spine of the scapula (Fig. 11) on its posterior surface. It passes laterally under the coracoacromial ligament and attaches to the greater tuberosity of the humeral head (Fig. 12). The greater tuberosity of the humerus is located lateral to the bicipital groove. The supraspinatus muscle is innervated by the suprascapular nerve C_4, C_5, C_6.

The *infraspinatus muscle* originates from the greater surface area of the infraspinatus fossa of the scapula located below the spine of the scapula. The muscle proceeds laterally to insert just below the attachment of the supraspinatus muscle on the greater tuberosity. The tendons of the supraspinatus, the infraspinatus, and the teres minor merge into a conjoined tendon before attachment (Fig. 12). The infraspinatus muscle is also innervated by the suprascapular nerve C_4, C_5, C_6.

The *teres minor muscle* arises from the lateral portion of the axillary border of the scapula (Fig. 11) and passes laterally and upward to insert on the humerus immediately below the infraspinatus, on the greater tuberosity. The teres minor receives a branch of the axillary nerve as it proceeds to the deltoid muscle, C_5 and C_6.

The *subscapularis muscle* (Fig. 13) is the most anterior and the most medial muscle of the cuff. It originates from the entire anterior

12

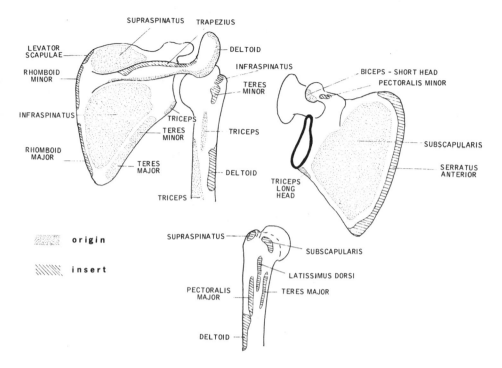

FIGURE 11. Sites of muscular origin and insertion upon the scapula and the humerus. All the muscles that perform shoulder girdle function are shown here. The stippled areas indicate the places from which the muscles originate, and the hatched areas represent spots upon which the muscles or their tendons insert.

(thoracic) surface of the scapula and proceeds laterally to attach to the lesser tuberosity of the head of the humerus. The lesser tuberosity is located just medial to the bicipital groove (see Figs. 7 and 9). The subscapularis muscle passes in front of the shoulder joint and is separated from the neck of the scapula by a bursa. This bursa (see Fig. 5) is a pouching of the synovial cavity of the shoulder joint. The muscle receives its nerve supply from the upper and lower subscapular nerves C_5 and C_6.[9]

There is an opening in the anterior portion of the cuff insertion upon the humerus, located between the supraspinatus muscle and the subscapularis muscle, through which the biceps tendon, its sheath, and an invagination of the synovial cavity pass. This opening is reinforced by the coracohumeral ligament (see Fig. 8), a ligament that proceeds from the coracoid process and fuses into the anterior superior aspect of the glenohumeral capsule. There is further reinforcement by the *transverse humeral ligament* (see Fig. 5) that holds the biceps tendon in

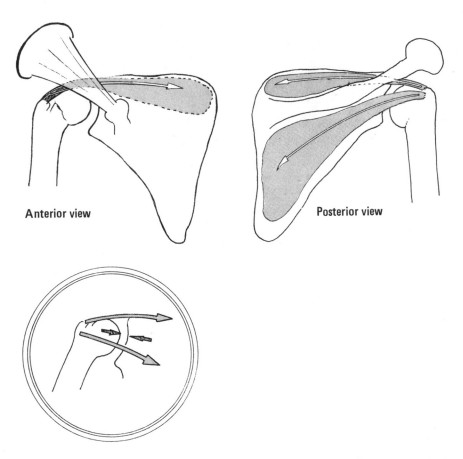

FIGURE 12. The supraspinatus muscle and the infraspinatus muscle. *Anterior view*: The supraspinatus muscle originates from the supraspinatus fossa of the scapula and passes laterally under the coracohumeral ligament to attach upon the greater tuberosity of the humerus. *Posterior view*: The infraspinatus muscle originates from the infraspinatus fossa and inserts upon the greater tuberosity just below the insertion of the supraspinatus tendon. The combined action of these two muscles (*insert*) brings the head of the humerus against the glenoid fossa in a slightly "downward" direction.

the biceps groove. The cuff's tendinous insertion is a conjoined tendon of all four cuff muscles: the supraspinatus, infraspinatus, teres minor, and the subscapularis (see Fig. 9).

When tears occur in the cuff, they usually occur longitudinally in the anterior portion of the cuff between the supraspinatus tendon and the coracohumeral ligament at the *critical zone*. This critical zone (Fig. 14) is the region of maximal tensile strength and is the area of vascular anastamosis between the osseous vessels (arteries) and the muscular vessels.

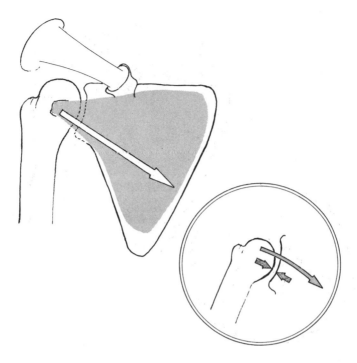

FIGURE 13. The subscapularis muscle. The subscapularis muscle originates from the entire anterior surface of the scapula (see Fig. 11), the surface that glides against the thoracic wall. The muscle extends laterally and attaches to the lesser tuberosity of the humerus. Its tendon is the most medial of those forming the "cuff." Its action is to pull the head of the humerus into the glenoid fossa and slightly downward.

The critical zone is so called because it is the site of degeneration and cuff tear is usually relatively ischemic. When the arm is dependent, hanging at the side, the cuff is under traction tension which obliterates or compresses the blood vessels. When the arm is actively abducting, the cuff muscles, especially the supraspinatus, are contracting and thus placing traction upon the conjoined tendon. Either during activity or during dependency the critical zone is ischemic. It is apparent that in an average 24 hours of normal activity there is ischemia during 12 to 18 hours. Only during recumbency is the cuff hyperemic. This may explain why symptoms occur at night (Fig. 15) (see Chapter 2).

The *deltoid muscle* (Fig. 16) arises anteriorly from the clavicle, laterally from the acromion, and posteriorly from the spine of the scapula (see Fig. 9), and passes down in front of, lateral to, and behind the shoulder glenohumeral joint. The fibers attach to the anterior lateral area of the middle third of the humerus. The basic action of deltoid

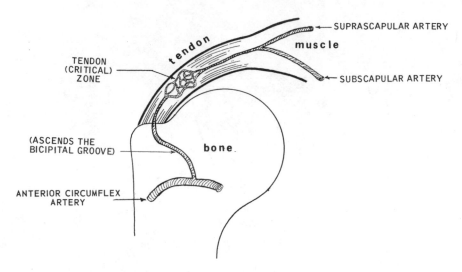

FIGURE 14. Circulation of the tendons of the cuff: the "critical zone." The tendons of the "cuff" have a highly vascular zone at the anastomosis of the muscular vessels and the osseous vessels. This "critical zone" is the portion with the greatest tensile strength and is also the area that accumulates the calcium deposits; thus it is the site of cuff ruptures. This zone is graphically shown, and the contributing vessels are identified.

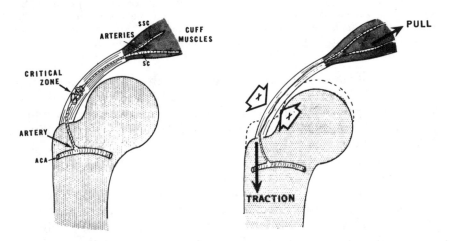

FIGURE 15. Blood circulation. *Left*: Circulation to the rotator cuff. The arterial branch from the anterior circumflex artery (ACA) enters from the bone. The suprascapular (SSC) and the subscapular (SC) branches merge to enter from the muscle. The critical zone of the tendon is an anastomosis which is patent when the arm is supported and inactive. *Right*: Traction upon the cuff from the dependent arm or from pull of the contracting cuff muscle elongates the tendon and renders the critical zone (*arrows*) relatively ischemic.

16

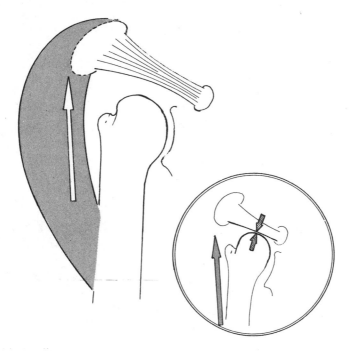

FIGURE 16. The deltoid muscle and its isolated function. The deltoid muscle originates from the inferior aspect of the spine of the scapula and the protruding acromial process (see Fig. 11). By its attachment into the humeral shaft, it has a direction of pull as depicted by the arrow in the large figure. Its isolated action shown in the circle is that of elevation, impinging the head of the humerus directly up under the coracoacromial arch. As the head of the humerus is rotated, depressed, and adducted into the glenoid fossa by the other cuff muscles, the deltoid becomes a powerful abductor.

contraction is elevation of the humerus along a line parallel to the humerus and tends to force the humeral head up against the coraco-acromial ligament (see insert, Fig. 15). When working in harmony with the cuff muscles, the middle (lateral) fibers of the deltoid abduct the arm in the coronal plane. The anterior deltoid fibers forward flex in the sagittal plane while slightly internally rotating the humerus. The posterior fibers extend the humerus posteriorly in the sagittal plane and externally rotate the humerus (Fig. 17). The deltoid muscle is innervated by the axillary nerve (C_5 and C_6).

GLENOHUMERAL MOVEMENT

Movement of the humeral head upon the glenoid fossa of the scapula is intricate in that the greater articular surface of the humerus, the male portion of the joint, is larger in area and is less convex than the glenoid fossa, the female portion of the joint. Glenohumeral

17

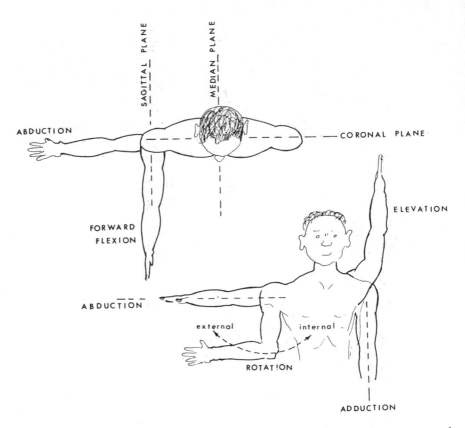

FIGURE 17. The planes of arm movement, indicating the direction of movement and the planes of movement in relation to the body. The body is viewed from above and from the front. All arm planes are related to these two body positions.

movement is a *gliding* of two incongruous surfaces. Abduction of the arm in the coronal plane is possible only by depression of the humerus to pass under the coracoacromial arch (Fig. 18).

Glenohumeral movement requires simultaneous abduction of the arm with depression of the humeral head. This complex movement occurs by coordinated action of the musculotendinous cuff muscles and the deltoid muscle. This motion is a part of the *scapulohumeral rhythm*.

The deltoid muscle, by virtue of its attachment from the inferior surface of the protruding acromial process and its attachment to the lateral portion of the upper third of the humerus, elevates the humerus along the line of the humeral shaft to butt the head of the humerus against the coracoacromial hood (see Fig. 16).

This upward movement of the head of the humerus must be in-

18

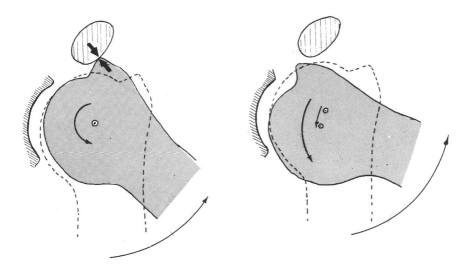

FIGURE 18. Glenohumeral movement of arm abduction. The incongruity of the articular surface of the head of the humerus and the surface of the glenoid fossa is shown. *Left*: The greater tuberosity of the humerus impinging upon the coracoacromial ligament if rotation is not accompanied by depression of the humerus. *Right*: Simultaneous depression and rotation in a gliding motion permitting the greater tuberosity to pass under the coracoacromial hood during arm abduction.

clined toward the glenoid fossa and simultaneously rotated downward to permit the greater tuberosity to pass under the coracoacromial ligament. This permits the arm to abduct to the horizontal position. The movement of rotation and fixation of the head of the humerus into the glenoid fossa is performed by the action of the cuff muscles.

Of the cuff muscles the supraspinatus arises from the supraspinatus fossa of the scapula and passes under the coracoacromial hood to attach upon the greater tuberosity and pulls the head of the humerus into the glenoid fossa. As its line of pull is slightly above the center of rotation (Fig. 19), it exerts rotatory motion of the head of the humerus. This rotation is considered by some to be minor,[10] but it is sufficient to place the humerus into adequate abduction to permit the deltoid to function. By pulling the head of the humerus horizontally, it also fixes the head into the glenoid fossa. When viewed superiorly, the line of pull is behind the linear axis of rotation of the humerus; thus the supraspinatus muscle also *externally rotates the humerus*. This latter action is important in the thorough motion required to place the arm overhead.

Early studies of kinesiology maintained that the supraspinatus initiated and acted during the first degrees of abduction with its maximum activity exerted at 100° of abduction. This has been disproven.[11]

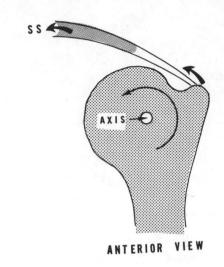

ANTERIOR VIEW

SUPERIOR VIEW

FIGURE 19. Function of the supraspinatus muscle. The anterior view shows supraspinatus function abducting the arm in the coronal plane. Viewed superiorly, this muscle externally rotates the arm.

Electromyographic studies have shown the supraspinatus to *act during the entire abduction* of the arm in the coronal plane. The function of the supraspinatus is a quantitative one. Paralysis of the supraspinatus muscle by a selective nerve block permits the arm to move through full range with minimal diminution of strength and endurance.[12]

In summary, the supraspinatus muscle acts in conjunction with the other cuff muscles during glenohumeral movement to bring the head into the glenoid fossa, exerting minimal rotatory action.

The remaining cuff muscles, the infraspinatus, subscapularis, and the teres minor, by their origin and insertion, have more of a downward pull and thus depress the head of the humerus in a downward rotatory direction. In addition to being termed *cuff* muscles, they are also called *short rotators* (Fig. 20). The subscapular muscle originates from the entire thoracic surface of the scapula and inserts into the lesser tuberosity of the humerus, having a similar action to the other

20

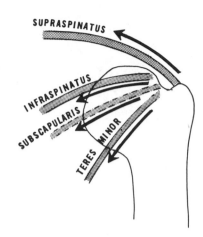

FIGURE 20. Rotator cuff mechanism. The supraspinous (supraspinatus) muscle pulls the head of the humerus into the glenoid and slightly rotates the humerus into abduction. The infraspinous (infraspinatus) muscle also rotates the head and slightly pulls it down. The teres minor muscle pulls in a more downward direction. The subscapular (subscapularis) muscle pulls the head into the glenoid, but its main rotatory action is to internally rotate the humerus about its longitudinal axis.

short rotators. The combined action of the cuff muscles pulls the humeral head into the glenoid fossa, depresses and rotates the head, fixes it there, and assists the deltoid in its abduction action (Figs. 21 and 22).

The active movement of the humerus at the glenohumeral joint differs from its passive range and is influenced by rotation of the humerus. The arm can be abducted *passively* to 120° with movement exclusively at the glenohumeral joint. After 120°, abduction is blocked by the humerus impinging upon the acromial process and the coracoacromial ligament. *Active* abduction is possible only to 90°, after which active abduction is possible only with simultaneous rotation of the humerus that permits the greater tuberosity of the humerus to pass posteriorly to the acromial process.

Only 60° of abduction is possible with the humerus in internal rotation, due to the fact that the humerus, in internal rotation, impinges much earlier upon the coracoacromial ligament than it does in external rotation (Fig. 23). This explains the limited shoulder abduction in patients who have a limited humeral rotation as a result of surgical repair of recurrent shoulder dislocations.

Since the arm can be abducted and elevated fully overhead, an arc of 180°, an additional 60° to the active 90° and passive 120° occurring at the glenohumeral joint must occur. This motion results from rotation of the scapula, adding an additional 60° to overhead elevation of the arm. The combined movement of the humerus upon the scapula at the glenohumeral joint and the scapula upon the thorax, in its simultaneous synchronous movement, conforms to the well-established *scapulohumeral rhythm.*[1]

Before discussing this total arm movement, the scapular phase of the rhythm requires evaluation.

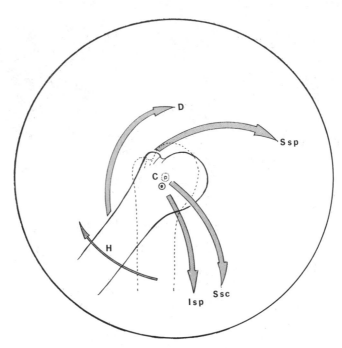

FIGURE 21. Combined cuff and deltoid action upon the glenohumeral articulation. Abduction of the humerus along the plane H is the result of combined action of the supraspinatus (Ssp) adducting the head into the fossa; the infraspinatus and subscapularis (Isp and Ssc) adducting and depressing the head; and the deltoid (D) acting as an abductor when working with these cuff muscles. The center of rotation (C) lowers during this downward gliding motion.

SCAPULAR MOVEMENT

The scapula moves in a gliding manner upon the thoracic wall at the thoracoscapular articulation. Movement occurs at the distal end of the clavicle, the acromioclavicular joint, by virtue of motion and rotation of the clavicle. Motion of the scapula is primarily produced by two muscles, the trapezius and the serratus anterior.

The broad fan-shaped trapezius muscle acts as three muscles (Fig. 24). The upper fibers of the trapezius originate from the ligamentum nuchae in the lower cervical region, the posterior spinous processes of the cervical spine, and the upper thoracic spine. They radiate laterally and downward to attach to the upper margin of the medial and central portion of the scapular spine.[13,14] The action of the upper trapezius pulls the scapula upward and causes inward pivoting about the acromioclavicular joint.

The middle fibers originate from the spinous processes of the upper thoracic vertebrae, proceed laterally, and attach to the medial border

22

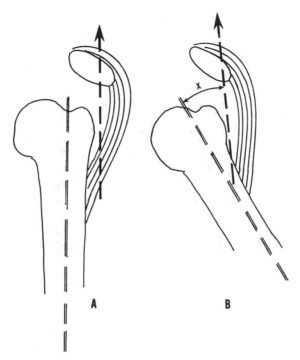

FIGURE 22. Abduction angle of deltoid. A. With the arm dependent, the deltoid line of pull is along the line of the humerus and thus elevates the arm up against the acromion. B. With slight abduction of the humerus the angle of the deltoid changes its pull to abduction of the arm.

of the scapular spine. These middle fibers principally "fix" the scapula during abduction of the arm. They must relax during forward flexion of the arm-shoulder in the sagittal plane (see Fig. 17).

The lower fibers of the trapezius originate from the spinous processes of the lower thoracic vertebrae and attach to the medial portion of the spine of the scapula. The isolated function of these fibers pulls the medial border of the spine of the scapula *down* and *in*. The combined action of the upper and lower trapezius fibers rotates the scapula around the axis center of the acromioclavicular joint, depressing the vertebral border, and elevating the glenoid fossa on the outer portion. The trapezius is supplied by the spinal accessory nerve (XI).

The serratus anterior is the other major muscle acting to rotate the scapula. This broad muscle originates from the upper eight ribs of the anterolateral chest wall, anterior to the scapula, and runs posteriorly to insert upon the medial (vertebral) border of the scapula. The heaviest fibers attach upon the inferior border. The serratus is located in the

23

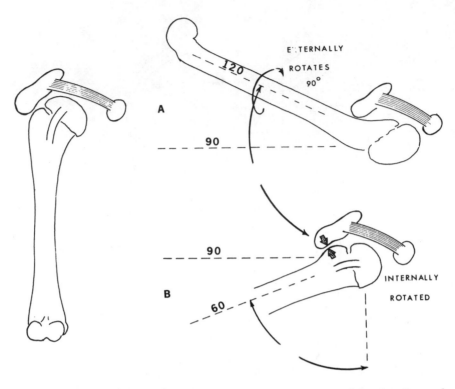

FIGURE 23. Influence of humeral rotation upon abduction range of the glenohumeral joint. *A.* Active abduction is possible to 90°, and an additional 30° can be gained passively if the humerus rotates externally approximately through a 90° arc. This abduction range of 120° is possible because the rotation allows the greater tuberosity to pass behind the acromion. *B.* With the arm internally rotated, the greater tuberosity impinges against the coracoacromial arch and blocks abduction at 60°.

scapulocostal joint space between the scapula and the rib cage. Its line of pull moves the scapula forward and, because it acts below the axis of the acromioclavicular joint, acts as a rotator. The serratus muscle is innervated by the long thoracic nerve formed by the anterior branches of the roots of C_5, C_6, and C_7 (primarily C_6) before they enter the brachial plexus.

The combined action of the upper trapezius, the lower trapezius, and the serratus causes rotation of the scapula about the pivotal point of the acromioclavicular joint and elevates the glenoid fossa.

Other muscles that act upon the scapula but are not involved in the scapulohumeral rhythm can be mentioned briefly. Under the trapezius are three muscles that attach to the vertebral border of the scapula: the levator scapula, the rhomboid major, and the rhomboid minor (Fig. 25). The levator scapula originates from the cervical trans-

24

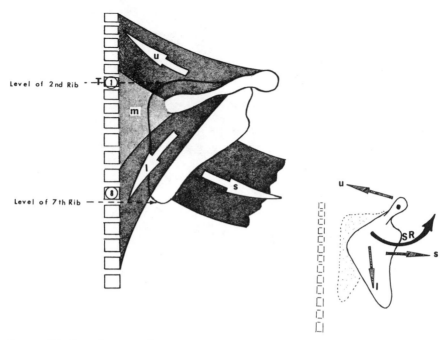

Level of 2nd Rib

Level of 7th Rib

FIGURE 24. Scapular musculature: rotators. The scapular muscles forming the rotator phase of the scapulohumeral rhythm are shown with the upper trapezius fibers elevating the outer border of the spine, the lower fibers of the trapezius depressing the medial border of the spine, and the serratus pulling the lower portion of the scapula forward from its position under the blade. The combined action moves the scapula in orbit around the acromioclavicular center of rotation (u, m, and l = upper, middle, and lower trapezius; s = seratus anterior; SR = scapular rotation).

verse processes and proceeds downward and laterally to attach to the superior angle of the scapula. The rhomboid minor is located immediately below the levator, originates from the lower cervical vertebra, and attaches to the vertebral border of the scapula at the level of the scapular spine. The rhomboid major, much broader than the above muscles, originates from the upper thoracic vertebrae and inserts into the remainder of the vertebral border of the scapula. They elevate the medial aspect of the scapula and cause downward rotation of the glenoid fossa by virtue of the rotation around the acromioclavicular pivotal point. These three muscles receive their nerve supply from C_5 through the dorsal scapular nerve.

Downward movement of the glenoid fossa is aided also by the action of the pectoralis major and the latissimus dorsi muscles acting upon the scapula indirectly through their attachments upon the humerus.

The pectoralis major has an extensive origin: from the sternal half of

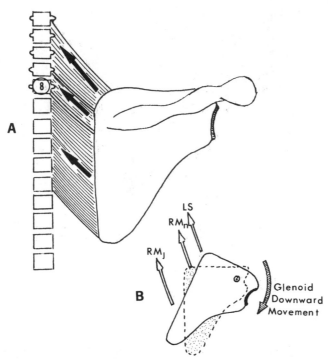

FIGURE 25. A. Downward rotators of the scapula. B. The muscles acting upon the scapula directly to cause downward rotation of the glenoid fossa are the levator scapulae (*upper arrow*), the rhomboid minor (*middle arrow*), and the rhomboid major (*lower arrow*).

the clavicle, the sternum and costal cartilages of the second to the seventh rib, and the fascia of the abdominal muscles (Fig. 26). It inserts into the crest of the greater tuberosity and downward along the humerus several inches. It is innervated by the medial and lateral thoracic nerves. Its function is primarily to pull the arm down from an overhead forward position, adducting the arms when held in front of the body, and internal rotation of the humerus.

The latissimus dorsi is the broadest muscle of the back and thoracic region. It originates from the spinous processes of thoracic 6 downward to the crest of the ilium. It inserts to the crest of the lesser tuberosity of the humerus. In its action it depresses the arm downward and internally rotates it.

The musculature acting upon the clavicle also effects scapular motion and will be discussed later.

SCAPULOHUMERAL MOVEMENT

Abduction elevation of the arm in the coronal plane, from de-

26

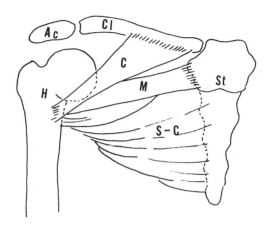

FIGURE 26. Pectoralis major. The pectoralis major has three laminae: clavicular (C), manubrial (M), and a sternocostal (S-C) bundle. All form the pectoralis muscle but are considered to have slightly separate functions.

pendency at the side of the body until fully extended overhead, with palms facing each other, is a smooth, synchronous motion involving every component of the shoulder girdle complex. Motion must be smooth and effortless, requiring full range of motion at each joint and well-coordinated muscle balance. *The normal composite movement is stressed because knowledge and recognition of the slightest imbalance and restriction must be recognized to evaluate the pain producing impairment of the shoulder.*

The smooth, integrated movement of the humerus, the scapula, and the clavicle has been well termed the "scapulohumeral rhythm" by Dr. E. A. Codman, whose book, *The Shoulder*, is a monumental study.[1]

Of every 15° of abduction of the arm, 10° occurs at the glenohumeral joint, and 5° from rotation of the scapula upon the chest wall. This 2:1 ratio of humerus to scapula exists throughout the entire abduction range in a smooth, rhythmic pattern (Fig. 27). To reiterate, the scapula can rotate 60°; the humerus, 90° actively and 120° passively.

The scapula rotates to maintain mechanical stability of the glenohumeral joint and efficiency of the deltoid muscle. The deltoid, as all muscles, has greatest efficiency at its *rest length* (Fig. 28), the point midway between its extremes of motion. The deltoid is at rest length when the arm is dependent at the side. Abduction shortens the muscle, and by 90° abduction with no scapular rotation, the extreme of contraction is reached. The deltoid then is barely able to support the arm. Scapular rotation maintains optimum deltoid length throughout abduction.

Full overhead elevation requires little or no deltoid support if the scapula has fully rotated. At this point the glenoid fossa is directly under the head of the humerus. Had there been no scapular rotation,

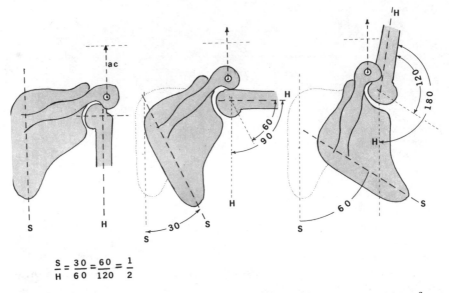

$$\frac{S}{H} = \frac{30}{60} = \frac{60}{120} = \frac{1}{2}$$

FIGURE 27. Scapulohumeral rhythm. The scapula and the humerus at position of rest with the scapula relaxed and the arm dependent, both at position 0°. The abduction movement of the arm is accomplished in a smooth, coordinated movement during which for each 15° of arm abduction 10° of motion occurs at the glenohumeral joint and 5° occurs due to scapular rotation upon the thorax. The humerus (H) has abducted 90° in relation to the erect body, but this has been accomplished by a 30° rotation of the scapula and a 60° rotation of the humerus at the glenohumeral joint, a ratio of 2:1. *Right*: Full elevation of the arm: 60° at the scapula and 120° at the glenohumeral joint.

the humerus could shear out of the glenoid fossa. This is a mechanism of shoulder dislocation.

Scapulohumeral movement at the glenohumeral joint and the scapulothoracic joint has been highlighted with "motion around the axis of the acromioclavicular joint." This joint and the sternoclavicular joint play a vital role in total arm motion.

ACROMIOCLAVICULAR AND STERNOCLAVICULAR JOINTS

The acromioclavicular joint is a plane joint connecting the outer end of the clavicle with its convex facet to the anterior medial portion of the acromial process. A fibrocartilaginous ring that resembles an intra-articular meniscus may exist. At the age of 2 years no joint space exists; the acromion and the clavicle are connected by a fibrocartilaginous bridge. At the age of 3 years, a joint space appears consisting of two synovial cavities, one at the end of the clavicle, the other at the acromial end, with an interposed *disk* between them (Fig. 29).

The disk becomes meniscoid by the second decade, and the articu-

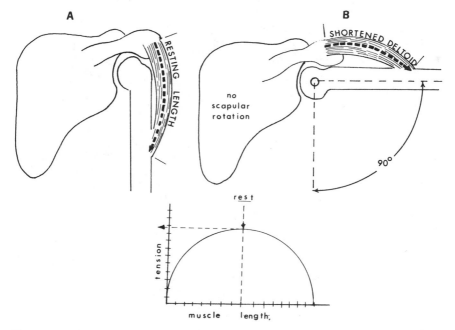

FIGURE 28. Deltoid action upon the glenohumeral joint. The mechanical efficiency afforded the deltoid action upon abduction of the humerus by the simultaneous rotation of the scapula is shown in the length-tension relationship upon muscle. Muscle efficiency is greatest at rest length and diminishes upon shortening. In the abducted arm without scapular rotation, the deltoid shortens to a length of less tension (B). Simultaneous scapular rotation keeps the deltoid at rest length (A).

lar surfaces of the acromion and the clavicle become smooth and glistening. After the second decade the disk and the articular surfaces undergo rapid degenerative changes that are marked by the fourth decade.[15]

The acromioclavicular joint has a weak, relaxed capsule that is reinforced by strong superior and inferior acromioclavicular ligaments that prevent posterior displacement of the clavicle upon the acromion.

The clavicle is firmly attached to the scapula by the coracoclavicular ligament (see Fig. 2). Two resilient fascicles, each called a ligament, form the coracoclavicular ligament: the lateral *trapezoid* and the medial *conoid* ligaments. The manner of attachment of these ligaments prevent the scapula from rotating about the acromioclavicular joint and, by its "strut" shape, maintains a constant relationship of the scapula to the clavicle (Fig. 30).

The coracoclavicular ligament, by its attachments in a strut shape was once considered instrumental in holding the scapula away from the chest wall and giving stability to the acromioclavicular joint. This

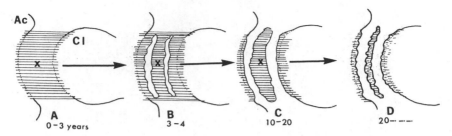

FIGURE 29. Evolution of the acromioclavicular disk (meniscus). A. From birth to age 2 a fibrocartilage bridge joins the acromion to the clavicle (Ac to Cl) with no joint space. B. From age 3 to 4, cavities form to either side of what will become the meniscus (x). C. In the first and second decades the meniscus is already beginning thinning and fibrillation, which increases rapidly from age 20 on. D. In the sixth decade the meniscus may be completely gone.

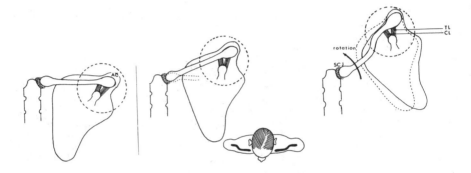

FIGURE 30. Action of the coracoclavicular ligaments upon the acromioclavicular joint. The coracoclavicular ligament attaches the scapula to the clavicle. It is divided into two resilient fascicles termed the trapezoid ligament and the conoid ligament. From the coracoid they proceed upward and laterally to attach onto the undersurface of the clavicle. Elevation of the clavicle without rotation maintains a constant relationship of the scapula to the clavicle. The rotation of the scapula depresses the coracoid and thus rotates the clavicle about its long axis. The left drawing depicts the scapula at rest with the coracoclavicular ligaments viewed through the sagittal axis (*dotted circle*). The middle drawing shows abduction of the clavicle along the coronal plane without rotation. The right drawing shows full elevation of the clavicle, still displaying an unchanged relationship of the scapula to the clavicle in this coronal plane. Motion through this range must occur at the sternoclavicular joint (SCJ).

is now disproven by the retention of stability after severence of this ligament. Instability results *only* when there is severence of the coracoclavicular ligament *and* the superior acromioclavicular ligament.[16]

As the scapula rotates to elevate the glenoid fossa, it rotates the clavicle about its long axis through the attachment of the coracoclavicular ligaments to the outer end of the clavicle. The "crank" shape of the clavicle elevates the outer end with no change in the angle of

30

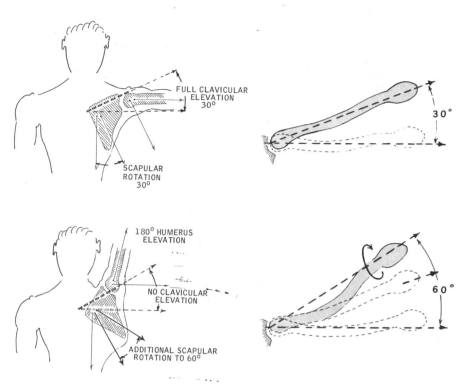

FIGURE 31. Scapular elevation resulting from clavicular rotation. The upper drawing shows the elevation of the clavicle without rotation to 30°. The remaining 30° of scapular rotation, which is imperative in full scapulohumeral range, occurs by rotation of the "crank-shaped" clavicle about its long axis.

elevation at the proximal sternoclavicular joint. Rotation of the clavicle occurs primarily in the overhead arm elevation above 90° abduction of the arm (Fig. 31). The first 30° of clavicular elevation occurs at the sternoclavicular joint. The next 30° of elevation is the result of rotation of the clavicle about its long axis.

The sternoclavicular joint is formed by the sternal end of the clavicle attaching to the superior lateral portion of the manubrium of the sternum and the cartilage of the first rib (Fig. 32). An articular disk between the sternum and the clavicle forms two joint spaces. Anterior and posterior sternoclavicular ligaments reinforce a loose fibrous capsule, and an interclavicular ligament connects the two clavicles. Stability of the joint is imparted by the costoclavicular ligament, a strong ligament that arises from the medial portion of the first rib and runs laterally and obliquely to attach into the undersurface of the clavicle (Fig. 32). This ligament stabilizes the clavicle against muscle action (Fig. 33) and acts as a fulcrum for all motions of the shoulder girdle.

31

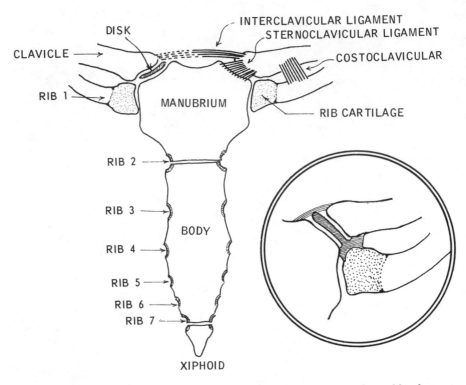

FIGURE 32. The sternoclavicular joint. The sternoclavicular joint is formed by the medial portion of the clavicle articulating upon the manubrium sterni and also with the cartilage end of the first rib. The ligaments that stabilize the joint are shown. The fibroelastic disk, or meniscus, is shown in the insert. In spite of marked movement at this joint in all shoulder girdle movements, arthritic changes are rare, mild, and rarely disabling.

The sternoclavicular joint, in spite of its plane joint surfaces, acts like a ball-and-socket joint, participating in all motions of the shoulder complex. In spite of its excess use, unlike the acromioclavicular joint, degenerative changes occur late in life and are mild with minimal functional impediment.[15]

COMPOSITE SHOULDER GIRDLE MOVEMENTS

Movement of the shoulder girdle requires smooth, effortless, synchronous movement of the glenohumeral joint and all the accessory joints. Each has been individually considered; now the composite movement can be related.

When the arm is raised in abduction, the humerus and the scapula move in a rhythm so that for every 15° of total abduction of the arm, 10° occurs at the glenohumeral joint, with a corresponding 5° of rotation of

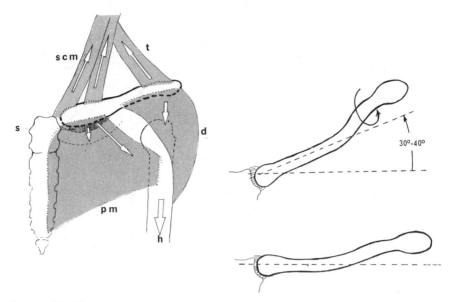

FIGURE 33. Muscles acting upon the clavicle. The major muscles acting upon the clavicle are shown, their direction of pull indicated by arrows: scm = sternocleidomastoid; t = trapezius; d = deltoid; s = subscapularis; and pm = pectoralis major. The gravity pull (h) of the arm itself is indicated as well. The muscles that act indirectly upon the clavicle are not shown.

the scapula. The humerus will complete its full possible abduction only if it externally rotates during elevation to permit the greater tuberosity to pass under and behind the coracoacromial ligament. Only 60° of humeral abduction is possible with the arm internally rotated. Only in the externally rotated position can the humerus abduct actively to 90°, and be passively abducted to 120°. Combined muscular action of the rotators and abductors performs this task (Fig. 34).

Full elevation of the arm overhead (180°) requires 60° of scapular rotation to alter the angle of the glenoid fossa upon which the humerus articulates. Scapular rotation results from the combined action of the trapezius and serratus muscles. Because the coracoclavicular ligaments prevent scapular rotation in the coronal plane, the scapula pivots about the acromioclavicular joint from rotation of the crank-shaped clavicle and elevation at the sternoclavicular joint.

Motion of the sternoclavicular joint is possible in all planes. The clavicle and the scapula are elevated by the trapezius and other accessory muscles that attach to the clavicle. For every 10° of arm elevation, 4° of the elevation occurs at the clavicle. There is varying elevation of the clavicle during the total arm elevation phase. Approximately 15° of clavicular elevation occurs during the first 30° of arm abduction, and

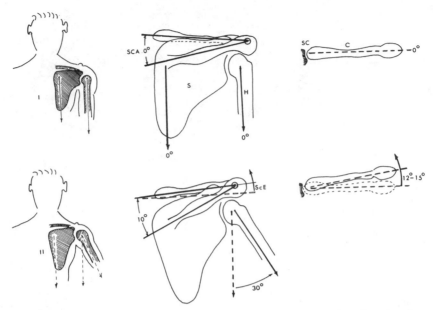

FIGURE 34. Accessory movement of the scapulohumeral rhythm other than the gleno-humeral movement. Movement of the arm through all phases of abduction involves all joints of the shoulder girdle in a synchronous manner.

Phase I: The resting arm: 0° scapular rotation (S); 0° spinoclavicular angle (SCA); 0° movement at the sternoclavicular joint (SC); no elevation of the outer end of the clavicle (C); no abduction of the humerus (H).

Phase II: Humerus abducted 30°: the outer end of the clavicle is elevated 12° to 15° with no rotation of the clavicle; elevation occurs at the sternoclavicular joint; some movement occurs at the acromioclavicular joint as seen by an increase of 10° of the spinoclavicular angle (SCA) formed by the clavicle and the scapular spine.

the clavicle has elevated to its final position as the arm reaches the horizontal level (90° abduction).

Half of the scapular rotation (30°) thus has been reached by clavicular elevation. The remaining 30° occurs by rotation of the crankshaped clavicle exerting pull on the coracoid process through the coracoclavicular ligaments. The clavicle rotates 45°, which raises the clavicle and its attached scapula an additional 30°. The greater part, if not all the rotation, occurs in the arm elevation above the horizontal position.

BICEPS MECHANISM

The biceps is anatomically and pathologically involved in the shoulder girdle, but its kinetics is unrelated to glenohumeral movement.

34

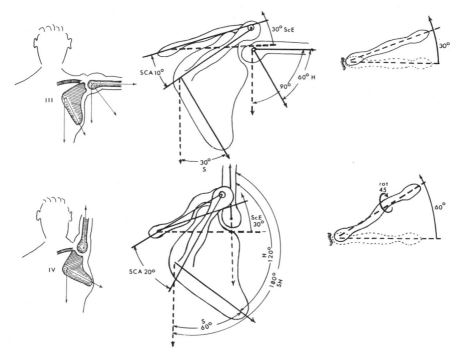

FIGURE 34 (continued).

Phase III : Humerus (H) abducted to 90° (60° glenohumeral, 30° scapular): the clavicle is elevated to its final position, 30°; no rotation of clavicle has occurred (all movement is at the sternoclavicular joint); no change in the SCA.

Phase IV: Full overhead elevation (SH = 180°; H = 120°; S = 60°): outer end of the clavicle has not elevated further (at the sternoclavicular joint), but the SCA has increased (to 20°). Because of the clavicle's rotation and its "cranklike" form, the clavicle elevates an additional 30°. The humerus through this phase has rotated, but this has not influenced the above degrees of movement.

The biceps brachii has two heads but a common tendon insertion into the tuberosity upon the inner aspect of the radius. The short medial head originates from the coracoid process. The long head originates from the superior lip of the glenoid fossa, proceeds laterally, and angles 90° at the bicipital groove of the humerus, to proceed downward to the common tendon (Fig. 35).

By its attachment on the ulnar side of the radius, its action is primarily supination of the forearm and secondarily elbow flexion. In the upper arm region the biceps assists the anterior deltoid in forward flexing the shoulder.

Motion of the biceps tendon does not occur in the unmoving bicipital groove. There is motion in the bicipital groove *only* when there is movement of the glenohumeral joint. Maximum downward movement

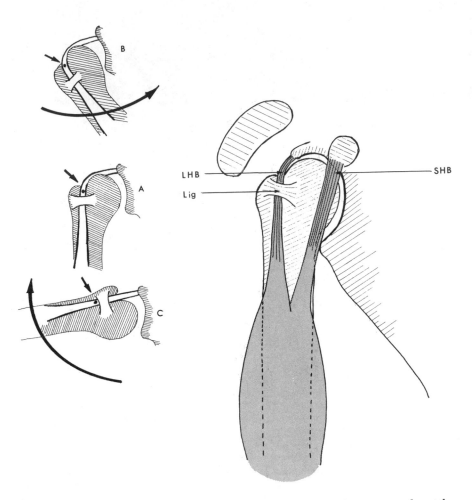

FIGURE 35. Biceps mechanism. The biceps brachii originates from two tendons: the short medial head, from the coracoid process; and the long head, from the superior rim of the glenoid fossa. The long head passes down into the bicipital groove in a fibrous sheath between the tendons of the subscapularis and the supraspinatus tendon. The small drawings at left depict the movement of the humerus upon the biceps tendon. A. The dependent hanging arm. B. Arm adducted, internally rotated, and extended, causing the ligament (*dot*) to move away from the transverse humeral ligament. C depicts the downward movement of the ligament (*dot*) below the transverse humeral ligament when the arm is abducted, externally rotated, and flexed forward.

of the tendon within the groove occurs when the arm is internally rotated and is elevated in the forward flexion movement. When the arm is flexed backward (extended) and abducted with the humerus externally rotated, the biceps tendon has the greatest upward movement within the groove (actually the biceps groove moves downward and thus the tendon glides upward). As any glenohumeral movement glides the tendon within the groove, free motion must exist to insure normal scapulohumeral movement. The bicipital mechanism is therefore essentially a passive action.

In severe deltoid paralysis, such as poliomyelitis, the biceps can become a "trick" abductor of the arm by the external rotation of the humerus. This lines up the belly of the biceps and the tendon in a direct line to the point of origin at the supraglenoid fossa; thus the biceps pull, with the humeral head held snugly in the fossa, weakly abducts the arm mechanically.

CHAPTER 2

Musculoskeletal Pain

The causes of pain in the shoulder, as enumerated in the outline on the following pages, are manifold. The most common cause of shoulder pain, constituting 90 percent of nontraumatic painful disabilities, is a degenerative tendinitis.[17] Among the names given to this condition are bursitis, pericapsulitis, adhesive capsulitis, and "frozen shoulder." The pathologic mechanism by which pain and dysfunction occur is more significant than the label, and by recognition of the abnormality of function that causes pain, rational treatment can be prescribed. The site of tissue pain can be determined by clinical examination (Fig. 36).

TENDINITIS: ATTRITION AND DEGENERATION

Man's upright posture and his daily activities are wearing on the supraspinatus tendons and the cuff-conjoined tendons. Gravity causes traction stress upon the capsule and tendons of the hanging arms, and movement of forward flexion and abduction cause friction and compression between the head of the humerus and the overlying coracoacromial ligament.

It has been noted that work requiring heavy lifting is not mandatory to cause shoulder pain from degeneration, but principally work with the hands at or above acromium height places a greater load upon the shoulders. This sustained position also causes sustained ischemia of the cuff and compresses the tendon between the greater tuberosity and the acromium[18] (see Fig. 15).

A progressive degeneration of the cuff has been noted in people unaware of pain or dysfunction.[2] In the fifth decade many cuffs are noted to be pulling away from their sites of insertion with the cuff showing signs of thinning and fibrillation. This thinning and degeneration are noted mostly within the "critical zone" (see Fig. 14), and the incidence of slight tears in later years becomes more marked. As

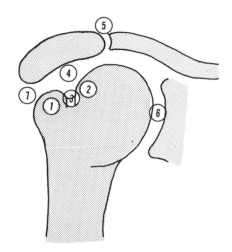

FIGURE 36. Sites of tissue pain: (1) greater tuberosity: attachment of supraspinatus tendon; (2) lesser tuberosity; (3) bicipital groove: tendon of long head of biceps; (4) subacromial bursa; (5) acromioclavicular joint; (6) glenohumeral joint and capsule; (7) subdeltoid bursa. (Modified from Steindler, A.: *The Interpretation of Pain in Orthopedic Practice.* Charles C Thomas, Springfield, Ill., 1959.)

the intensity of cuff degeneration becomes more apparent, some wearing away of the tuberosities of the humerus can also be noted (Figs. 37 and 38). This is evidently due to the deltoid action of elevation of the humerus up against the coracoacromial hood being unopposed by the depressing and rotating action of the cuff "rotators."

Absorption of the tuberosities must also find compression of the bicipital tendon as the bicipital groove becomes shallow and distorted, and even completely obliterated. The subacromial bursa (see Fig. 40) is also caught between these compressive pressures, and the bursal walls thicken and, when there is rupture of the tendon or invasion by calcium, become distended. The inferior surface of the acromion, from friction and pressure of the abutting humerus, becomes eburnated and thickened.

Aging must be considered a significant factor in degenerative tendinitis. Other factors, however, are also at play.

It was noted during the discussion on functional anatomy that in abduction of the arm the humeral head must be depressed within the glenoid fossa and glide downward to permit the greater tuberosity to pass under the coracoacromial arch. The posterior part of the arch, the acromion, is farther removed from the glenoid cavity than are the coracoid and the ligament (see Fig. 2). The greater tuberosity does not hit the acromion, but is constantly pressing against the ligament in everyday activities requiring elevation and abduction of the arm.[19] Almost every daily arm activity involves some degree of abduction.

During abduction of the arm internal rotation decreases the active and passive range of motion at the glenohumeral joint from 90° to 60° (see Fig. 18). A "round-shouldered" posture will depress the glenoid fossa and thus also depress the acromial arch and cause impingement

39

OUTLINE OF THE CAUSES OF PAIN FELT IN THE UPPER EXTREMITY

I. **Musculoskeletal**

  A. Degenerative
     1. Tendinitis, with or without calcific deposits
     2. Cuff tear, partial or complete

  B. Traumatic
     1. Fracture
     2. Dislocation
     3. Acromioclavicular separation
     4. Biceps tendon tear

  C. Inflammatory
     1. Rheumatoid arthritis
     2. Gout
     3. Infectious arthritis

  D. Tumors
     1. Bone
     2. Soft tissue

II. **Neurologic**

  A. Peripheral nerve
     1. Root (cervical)
       a. Spinal foraminal
         (1) Spondylosis
         (2) Herniated disk
         (3) Traumatic
           (a) Fracture
           (b) Dislocation
       b. Extramedullary tumors

     2. Brachial plexus
       a. Mechanical
         (1) Neurovascular bundle compression ("cervical dorsal outlet syndromes")
         (2) Scalene anticus syndrome
         (3) Cervical rib
         (4) Claviculocostal syndrome
         (5) Pectoralis minor syndrome

  b. Trauma
   (1) Traction or penetrating injuries
  c. Inflammatory
   (1) Brachial plexitis
  d. Tumors
   (1) Pancoast
   (2) Adenitis
 B. Central nervous system
  1. Intramedullary tumors
  2. Syringomyelia

III. Vascular

 A. Arterial
  1. Occlusive: acute and chronic
   a. Embolic
   b. Vasospastic
   c. Traumatic
   d. Atherosclerotic
  2. Aneurysm or fistula
 B. Venous
  1. Phlebitis
 C. Lymph
  1. Lymphedema

IV. Referred Visceral-Somatic Pain

 A. Cardiac
  1. Anginal pain
  2. Hand-shoulder syndrome
   a. Causalgia
 B. Gallbladder
 C. Diaphragmatic
 D. Ruptured viscus

V. Articular

 A. Degenerative
 B. Inflammatory
 C. Infectious
 D. Metabolic

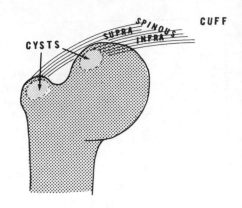

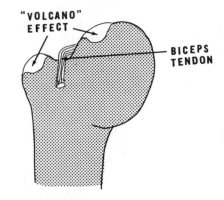

FIGURE 37. Roentgenographic changes in shoulder dysfunction: cysts in the tuberosities of the humerus. These are early x-ray evidence of attrition. With wear and tear, the tuberosities become eroded, causing a volcano appearance. The bicipital groove becomes shallow.

much sooner in arm motions. This can be verified by abducting the arms in the coronal plane to overhead position in the erect posture, then attempting the movement in a forced "slumped" posture. The latter will impede abduction markedly. It can be noted that the "slumped" posture internally rotates the arms, further impeding abduction.

Aging impairs joint range of motion because of the altered position of the scapula, and, in turn, because of the increased dorsal spinal kyphosis from dorsal disk degeneration. In the forward and backward lifting of the upper arm there is a decrease of 50° (from 240° in youth to 190° at age 70) and a similar decrease in abduction (166° in the young and 116° at age 70).[20] This slumped posture due to aging is also manifest in postural problems, occupational positions, and the postural depictions of the emotions (Fig. 39).[21]

42

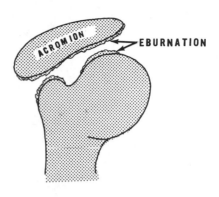

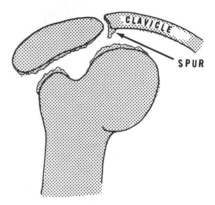

FIGURE 38. Stages of degeneration. *Top*: The tuberosities disappear and are replaced by eburnated bone. *Bottom*: In addition to hypertrophic change of the humeral head and the acromion, there are changes in the acromioclavicular joint, including spur formation.

CALCIFIC TENDINITIS

The pathogenesis and evolution of calcific tendinitis are shown in Figure 40.

The earliest microscopic changes are hyaline degeneration of the collagen in the tendon. There is disintegration of the nuclei and further degeneration of the tendon fibers which fibrillate, loosen, and ultimately separate. As they become pulverized between the grinding surfaces of the acromioclavicular ligament and the head of the humerus, they form small particles. When these particles are small, they are not visible in roentgenograms. They are said to be present in most people by age 35.[17]

This debris consists primarily of calcium salts in a highly vascular area,[22] contrary to the old notion that degenerative tendinitis occurs in an avascular tendon. In the dry state this powder casts a dense x-ray shadow. If the tendon is traumatized, the resultant hyperemia absorbs the calcium, forming a liquid, chalky material under pressure within

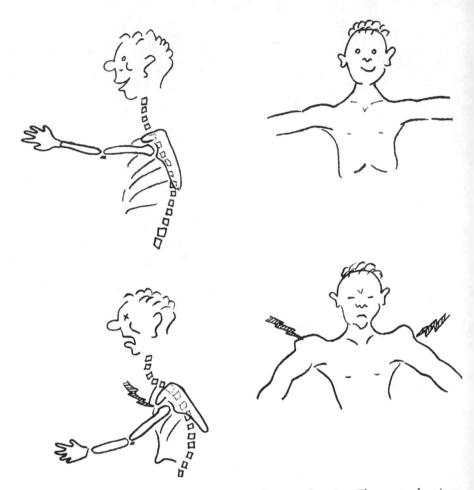

FIGURE 39. Postural effect upon glenohumeral range of motion. The upper drawings show the erect, "good" posture of the young: the forward elevation and the lateral abduction range of the arm is full and free; the coracoacromial ligament is elevated, and the humerus can do its corrective external rotation to allow the greater tuberosity to pass under the acromion. The lower drawings depict the dorsal kyphotic posture of the aged, the depressed individual, or the occupationally stressed person, in which the coraco-acromial hood is lowered and the arm is internally rotated. Both of these factors cause impingement of the humerus against the arch. Compression and attrition of the cuff tendons result.

the tendon. On x-ray the appearance fades into a translucency. The double arrows between the stages in Figure 40 indicate that many of these stages are reversible. Engorgement may be followed by "chalk" and conversely revert into the dry, "silent" inclusion. The "silent" phase may be composed of particles so small as to be invisible on x-ray.

44

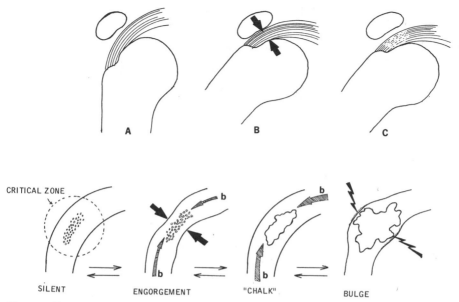

CRITICAL ZONE

SILENT   ENGORGEMENT   "CHALK"   BULGE

FIGURE 40. Natural sequence of calcific tendinitis. *A.* The relationship of the supraspinatus (cuff) tendon between the coracoacromial ligament and the head of the humerus. *B.* The repetitive pressure from daily use and abuse. *C.* The degenerative changes of the tendon in the "critical zone." The lower sequence follows the silent asymptomatic phase in the sequence steps to that of symptomatic "bulging." Compression from whatever external cause results in engorgement via the tendon circulation. The debris of the "silent" phase absorbs fluid, and the dry powder becomes chalk. Further irritation and engorgement cause the chalk to expand, or bulge. The double arrows signify that each phase is reversible.

The bulge phase presents a mechanical obstacle to smooth, pain-free abduction so that abduction, at approximately 70°, will impinge under the coracoacromial ligament. Pain will result from this increased tendon tension from compression. If the arm can be carried further in its abduction cycle, the bulge may pass beyond the ligament and become painless at 110°. Repeated abduction of the arm compresses this bulge further and increases the engorgement. Further increases of the bulge ensue, and a vicious circle results.

Rest or treatment may resolve this irritation and allow the inflammation to resolve. A return to "chalk" stage or the silent phase, can be expected. Increase of the bulge and concomitant engorgement will result in rupture of the calcific mass out of the tendon in the various directions and locations depicted in Figure 41.

The deposit may rupture superiorly and locate under the subdeltoid bursa. The ruptured deposit is frequently only partially evacuated (Fig. 41, parts 3 and 4); thus the relief of painful tension is temporary. It may recur repeatedly until there is complete evacuation in various

45

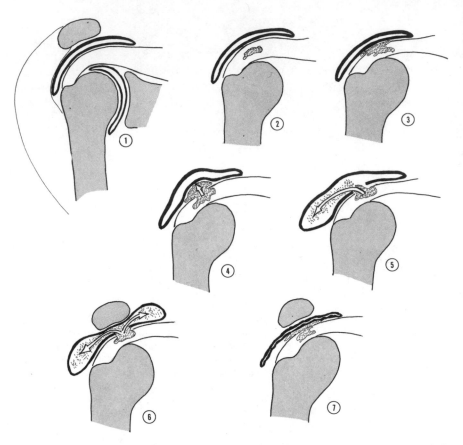

FIGURE 41. Evolution of the calcified tendinitis and formation of "bursitis." 1. The normal relationship of the supraspinatus tendon (cuff) to the coracoacromial arch and the head of the humerus; the intimate relationship of the subdeltoid bursa and the glenohumeral joint. 2. The site of calcium deposit in the cuff tendon. 3. The "bulging" calcium has been evacuated from the tendon into the subbursal space. 4. A partial evacuation into the subbursal space with much debris remaining within the tendon. 5. Tendon evacuates, with rupture into the subdeltoid bursa. 6. "Dumbbell" intrabursal invasion. 7. Adhesive bursitis in which there is thickening of the walls of the bursa and adhesion between the superior and inferior surfaces.

other manners or the overlying bursa becomes adherent and thickened (Fig. 41, part 7). The evacuated debris may work itself laterally and distally and repose under the deltoid insertion at the upper lateral aspect of the humerus, where it is no longer under tension nor an impediment to abduction.

The subbursal evacuation of the deposit may elevate the floor of the bursa and by pressure and irritation may rupture into the bursal sac. The rupture evokes acute, severe pain followed by a dull, deep aching, depending on the direction the calcium moves within the bursa. If the debris moves laterally and distally within the bursa (Fig. 41, part 5), the tenderness is felt at the lateral insertion of the deltoid, and the arm moves more freely under the coracoacromial ligament impingement. If the debris divides into a "dumbbell" form within the bursal sac, (Fig. 41, part 6) separated by the coracoacromial ligament, the arm will neither fully abduct nor adduct. It will be held in a partial abduction position (30° to 45°), resisting any movement.

The repeated bursal sac inflammation from persistent pressure may cause chronic thickening of the bursal lining, thickening of the bursal fluid, and adherence of the bursal walls; and an "adhesive pericapsulitis" results (see Fig. 43). This leads to a form of "frozen shoulder," when it is remembered that the superior wall of the bursa is adherent to the undersurface of the deltoid muscle and the inferior wall is adherent to the cuff. Other concepts of the "frozen shoulder" will be discussed later.

Erosion of the calcific mass inferiorly into the humerus is a possibility. This is not shown in Figure 41. This development is not usually visualized on x-ray study but is revealed at surgery when intractable pain requires surgical intervention.

In a brief summary, therefore, it may be assumed that over a long period of time, even normal use of the arm may produce considerable wear and tear to the cuff muscles and their tendons. Occupational factors, abuses of the arm, faulty posture, trauma, and emotional factors may hasten degenerative changes. Nature attempts to repair these tissue changes of damage by scar and ultimately by calcium deposit. So long as the deposit of debris remains *within* the tendon and under *no tension*, the shoulder is painless and unrestricted. Sudden injury precipitates the clinical picture of pain and impaired motion.

BURSITIS

Before proceeding further in the clinical discussion of tendinitis, calcific or noncalcific, "bursitis" merits discussion. This term is most frequently used when shoulder pain is considered.

Bursitis is rarely a primary condition. Most frequently it is secondary to degenerative lesions of the cuff and thus is a secondary phenomenon. The intimate relationship of the walls of the subdeltoid bursa, superiorly to the highly vascular and richly sympathetic nerve-supplied subdeltoid fascia and inferiorly inseparably adherent to the supraspinous portion of the cuff relates any pathology of the tendon to pathology of the bursa. The *subdeltoid bursa* is essentially the inner lining of the deltoid and the acromium and the outer layer of the cuff (Fig. 42). Filled with a small amount of fluid, any movement of the

47

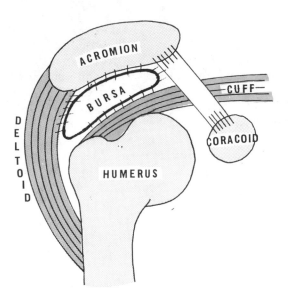

FIGURE 42. Subacromial bursa. The subdeltoid bursa is essentially the inner synovial lining of the deltoid muscle and the undersurface of the acromium. The outer layer of the supraspinatus portion of the cuff is the inner layer of the bursa. In any movement of the arm, the two layers of the bursa glide upon each other as the bursa deforms.

arm in abduction or forward flexion causes the two adjacent layers of the bursa to glide upon each other. Any adjacent inflammation of the tendon causes inflammation of the bursa. It is inconceivable that bursitis could exist without tendinitis and vice versa.

DIAGNOSIS

In a person who must be assumed to have a relative degree of cuff tendon degeneration, depending on age, posture, occupation, and psychological makeup, and who has previously been asymptomatic, onset of pain can occur after a particularly strenuous activity such as painting a ceiling or working in an awkward posture for long periods of time. Causes of acute precipitation of shoulder pain can include immobilization of the arm in a plaster cast for any reason, working on a tedious task in a slumped position, making sudden movements in an abnormal direction, or performing normal movements, but in a moment of fear, tension, or anxiety.

The adage of causation of musculoskeletal pain applies. *Pain can result in any of three conditions: (1) abnormal strain on a normal joint, (2) normal strain on an abnormal joint, or (3) normal stress upon a normal joint when the joint is unprepared and graded for that*

48

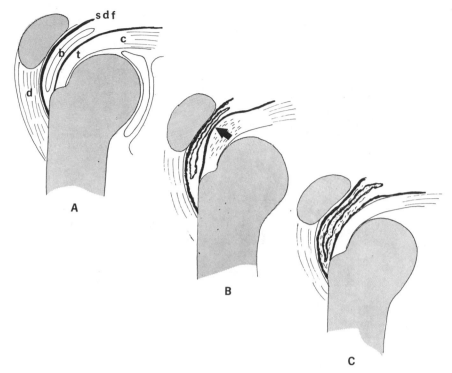

FIGURE 43. Acute tendinitis and inflammation of contiguous tissues. *A.* The tissues contained between the rotator cuff (c) and its tendons (t), and the subdeltoid fascia (sdf) lining the undersurface of the deltoid muscle (d). The subdeltoid fascia is rich in blood vessels and sympathetic nerves which originate in the stellate ganglia. Between the subdeltoid fascia and the fascia covering the cuff is loose connective tissue within which is located the subdeltoid bursa (b). *B.* Acute bulging of the tendon compresses and causes inflammation and swelling of the fascial tissues and the bursa. This is the acute mechanical phase during which there is severe pain and mechanical limitation of motion. *C.* The bulging of the tendon has subsided, but the resultant fascia and bursal inflammation persists, causing stiffness of the shoulder. *A* can go to *B* then to *C* and reverse through the entire phase back to *A.* The tendon remains frayed, and degenerative changes remain.

particular activity.[21] As has been considered in Chapter 1, the concept of a joint is a complex one. The movements of the glenohumeral joint and all other accessory joints elevate and abduct the total upper extremity in a smooth, effortless motion. The balance and synchronization are so accurate that the slightest disturbance in muscular activity, faulty joint direction or range, or external stress can upset the scapulohumeral rhythm. Pain, dysfunction, and limitation of motion can result.

Pain is the initial symptom and varies in intensity. The stress, the

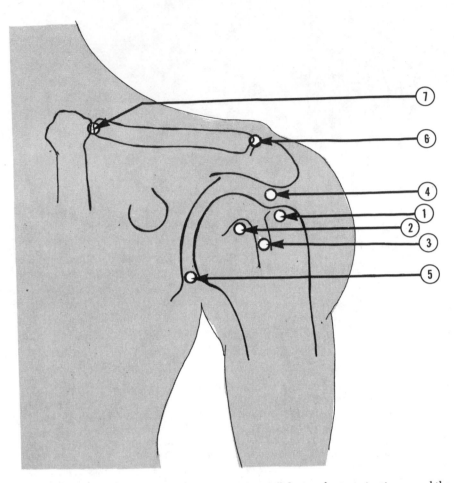

FIGURE 44. Trigger points. Palpable "trigger points" during the examination reveal the site of the pathology, corroborate the history, and indicate the type of therapy. 1. The greater tuberosity and the site of supraspinatus tendon insertion. 2. Lesser tuberosity, site of subscapularis muscle insertion. 3. Bicipital groove in which glides the bicipital tendon. 4. Site of the subdeltoid bursa. 5. Glenohumeral joint space. 6. Acromioclavicular joint. 7. Sternoclavicular joint.

degree of swelling of the tendon, and the pain threshold of the patient can alter the intensity of pain. Pain is usually localized in the shoulder region. In initial attacks it is localized in the anterior lateral aspect of the glenohumeral joint in the vicinity of the greater tuberosity and the overhanging acromial process. Associated local tenderness is frequent (Fig. 43).

Pain, from the onset, is associated with limitation, if not total prevention, of motion. Abduction is especially limited. Forward flexion

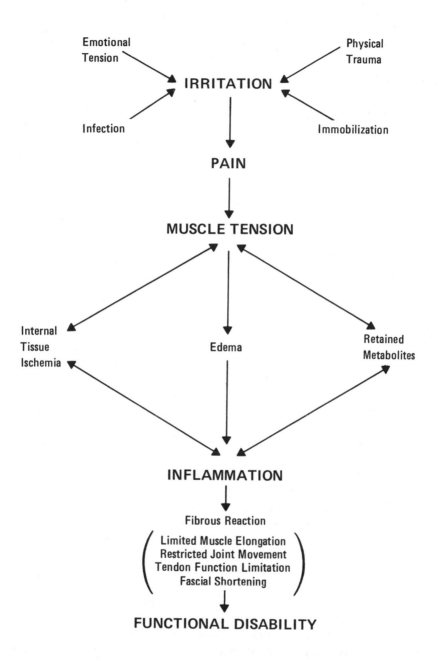

FIGURE 45. Mechanism by which irritation leads to functional disability.

and rotation also are usually markedly limited, with either active or passive motion causing an aggravation of pain. The reason for pain has already been noted. The offending swollen tendon contained within a narrow space is compressed between the moving humeral head and the overhanging acromial process and the coracoacromial ligament and arch.

As was depicted in Figure 44, the hanging dependent arm causes the critical zone of the conjoined cuff tendon to be ischemic, as does the contracting cuff in the abducting arm. In the resting arm the zone becomes hyperemic, especially when irritated. At this point the tendon is too swollen to pass between the greater tuberosity and the acromium.

The fact that the resting arm (i.e., the arm that is not dependent or actively abducting or forward flexing) allows the cuff to become hyperemic probably explains the frequency and severity of nocturnal pain in acute tendinitis.

"Shrugging" of the shoulder replaces smooth, effortless scapulo-humeral motion. "Shrugging" implies movement of the scapular phase of the rhythm without simultaneous glenohumeral movement; thus the scapula "shrugs" (elevates). The arm, limited at the gleno-humeral joint, does not abduct. External and internal rotation are equally limited and painful, but "shrugging" here is not noted as there is less rhythmical scapular associated movement in these particular movements. The glenohumeral movement, in external and internal rotation, is merely obstructed locally, and pain is felt locally. Movement is restricted at that joint.

Rest and treatment at this point may cause the acute phase to subside and full and pain-free motion to return. The swelling within the tendon and the inflammation of the contiguous tissues can abate, and movement between the humeral head and the overhanging arch resumes. The swelling that occurs in the peritendinous tissues, within the subdeltoid fascia, may persist and leave a relatively painless restricted movement, a "stiffness." This impaired scapulohumeral rhythm predisposes to further tendon irritation, degeneration, swelling, and recurrence of "acute" tendinitis. A recurrent vicious circle ensues. The pathomechanics sequence sets the rationale for proper treatment.

Should repeated irritation occur, the tendon may increase in size and may rupture its now liquid material out of the sheath to the sub-bursal area or into the bursal sac (see Fig. 41). The pain now is more severe and more constant, regardless of movement. This continuous, deep pain is caused by the constant tension within these tissues held within the confines of the narrow container. Any movement now is prohibited both by mechanical obstruction and by pain and protective

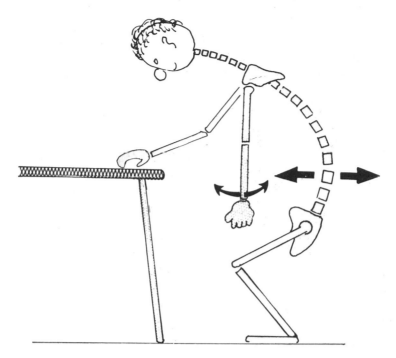

FIGURE 46. Pendular exercise. The patient bends forward, flexing the trunk to right angles. The involved arm is dangled without muscular activity of the glenohumeral joint. The body actively sways, thus passively swinging the dependent arm in forward flexion-extension, lateral swing, and rotation. The body can be supported by placing the other arm upon a table or chair. The arm is *passively* swung. No weight is held in the hand as this causes muscular contraction of the arm and the shoulder.

spasm. Restriction is in all ranges of glenohumeral motion, and the "shrugging" mechanism is total.

If the material ruptures outwardly and downward into the lower portion of the subdeltoid bursa, the pain and tenderness may be felt lower in the arm, at the lateral upper third of the humerus, where the deltoid inserts upon the humerus. Due to the residual subdeltoid fascial and bursal inflammation, "stiffness" of the glenohumeral joint remains, exhibiting a "stretch" type of pain.

TREATMENT

During the acute phase rest is desirable. A sling is frequently helpful. Ice packs, rather than heat, are indicated during the acute phase, which lasts for approximately 2 days. Heat appears to increase the engorgement of the inflamed tissues within the suprahumeral space. Ice decreases spasm, acts as a local cutaneous anesthetic, and has

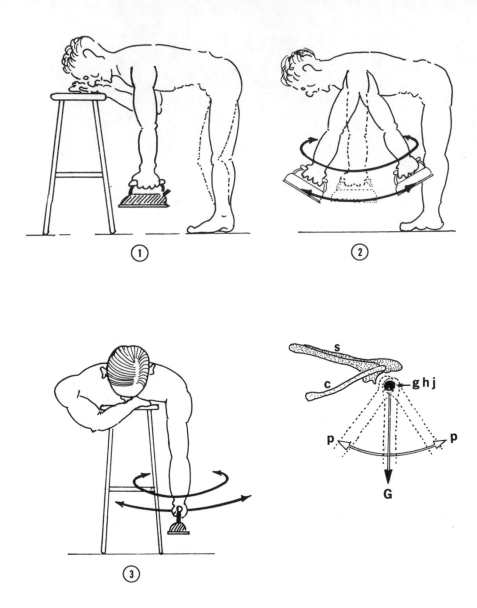

FIGURE 47. Active pendular glenohumeral exercise. 1. The posture to be assumed to permit the arm to "dangle" freely, with or without a weight. 2. The arm moves in forward and back sagittal plane, in forward and backward flexion. Circular motion in the clockwise and counterclockwise direction is also done in ever-increasing large circles. 3. The front view of the exercise showing lateral pendular movement actually in the coronal plane. The lower right diagram shows the effect of gravity (G) upon the gleno-humeral joint (ghj) with an immobile scapula (s). The p to p arc is the pendular movement.

reflex action in relieving pain.[23] It has been shown that intramuscular temperatures, at a depth of 3 cm, are not affected until after a 10-minute cooling period. A 20-minute period causes adequate, although not the final, cooling. Icing can be administered by means of a towel enclosing ice chips, ice in a rubber bag, or ethyl chloride spray. The spray, an explosive gas, carries some risks and is more difficult to self-administer.

Immobilization of the shoulder should never be prolonged. Immobilization, whether induced by the patient as a "fear of hurting" mechanism or by the iatrogenic factor in which the doctor or therapist does not limit the duration of immobilization, tends inevitably to fibrous reaction. The mechanism by which immobilization, along with factors of trauma, infection, or emotional tension, initiates fibrous reaction and functional disability is shown in Figure 45.

Immobilization fosters internal tissue ischemia, retention of metabolites, and edema. Since the major tissues about the shoulder are muscular and therefore for normal nutrition must contract and relax, be shortened and elongated, the mechanism of disability from immobilization is apparent. Immobilization, whether self-induced or medically advised, leads to disuse, which has been claimed to be a causative factor in pericapsulitis or "adhesive" capsulitis.[24,25] Disuse leads to muscular atrophy and to loss of capsular elasticity.

The limitation of motion of the shoulder is probably caused by proliferative inflammation of the soft-tissue components of the periarticular gliding tissues that ultimately lead to fibrosis. Immobilization entails circulatory disorders leading to ischemia and secondary metabolic changes of the connective tissue.

To prevent immobilization early in the treatment, active range of motion exercises should be insituted. "Early" means usually within the first week and more frequently within the first 4 days. Insofar as the motion of abduction-elevation causes impingement of the inflamed bursa and tendon between the acromial process and the greater tuberosity of the humerus, this maneuver should be avoided.

An antigravity exercise in which impingement is minimized and abduction is avoided, yet in which motion of the glenohumeral joint is achieved, is the Codman, or pendular, exercise. This exercise adds traction to the glenohumeral joint, stretches the capsule, avoids active abduction, and minimizes the "shrugging" scapular elevation imposed by gravity upon the erect posture.

As described by Codman, the pendular exercises are done passively with the arm dangling. No muscular activity of the shoulder is exerted. No weight is held actively in the hand, as any muscular contraction of the hand, wrist, or upper arm will cause a co-contraction of more proximal muscles. A weight held passively attached to the wrist may

55

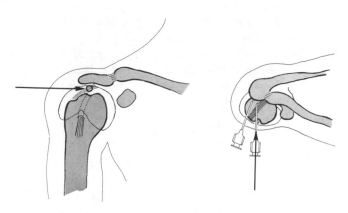

FIGURE 48. Technique of tendinitis-bursitis injection. *Left*: The anterior view depicts the site of entrance of the needle, as shown by the arrow. The palpating finger can feel the overhanging acromial process and the bicipital groove. Injection is just lateral to the sulcus at the greater tuberosity where the superspinatus tendon inserts. *Right*: Viewed from above, two directions of entrance are shown, with the arrow depicting that shown in the anterior view.

be utilized to cause more pendular motion and more traction at the shoulder. The arm is moved *passively* by the undulating body (Fig. 46).

The active pendular exercise is a modification of the Codman pendular exercise and is undertaken as soon as pain and restricted movement permits. The active pendular exercise is done in the same body position, but the arm is *actively* swung in the pendular planes (Fig. 47). A weight can now be held in the hand and be of increasing weight. All planes of movement are indicated: forward, sideways and circumduction, and with increasing amplitude of arc.

The exercise must be done properly. The patient bends forward at the waist to achieve a right angle trunk flexion. Slightly bent knees will decrease the low back and hamstring stretch pain. The head, rested upon a firm object and resting upon the other hand, permits relaxed movement and concentration upon the indicated movement of the involved shoulder.

In this position the dependent arm dangles vertically. Pendular motion is started (1) in a lateral medial plane ("out and in"); then (2) in a sagittal plane forward and backward (up and down with the body upright); then (3) in a gradually increasing circle; and finally (4) clockwise then counterclockwise. The use of an iron has been advocated as the weight since it is readily available in the home. A weight is frequently desirable as it adds traction to the dependent arm and widens the pendular cycle.

Movement must be consciously achieved at the glenohumeral joint,

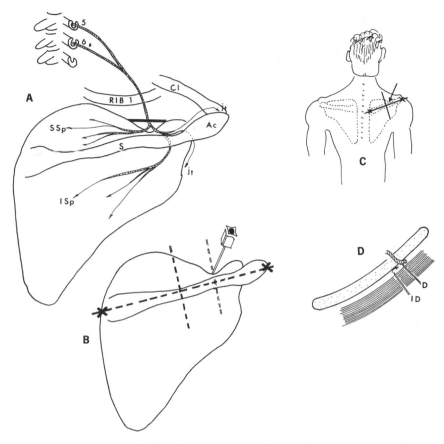

FIGURE 49. Suprascapular nerve block. *A*. The anatomy and course of the suprascapular nerve, originating from C_{5-6}. The motor nerve to the supraspinatus (SSp), and infraspinatus (ISp) and the sensory branches to the acromioclavicular joint and the shoulder joint (jt) are shown. *B,C*. Bisection of a line drawn along the scapular spine with the site of the groove and of needle insertion. *D*. The difference between direct nerve contact and indirect (ID) by infusion along the posterior portion of the scapula below the supraspinatus muscle.

with effort and thought directed to minimize scapular movement. The dependent arm adds traction, and the pendular movement causes range of motion at the glenohumeral joint in a manner that does not impinge the supraspinatus tendon.

As the range of motion increases and becomes less painful, heat can be applied, usually by the third day. Moist heat is preferable and may be applied by hot, moist towels kept warm by an electric pad or by chemical (hydrocollator) packs. The latter are more expensive, but they have the benefit of simplicity, more prolonged heat, and the

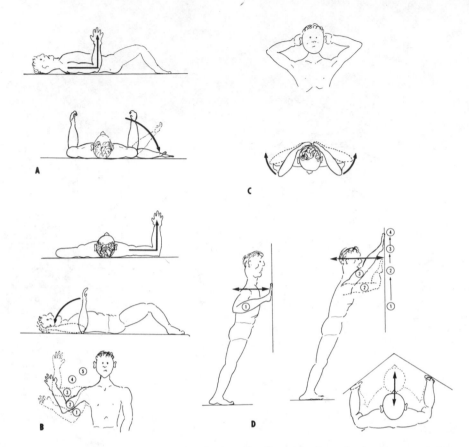

FIGURE 50. Exercises. *A.* Lying on back with elbows at the side, hands toward the ceiling. External rotation is attempted actively by the patient and passively by the therapist. Resistance may be applied when range permits. This exercise can be performed in the upright position against the wall. *B.* Similar exercise to *A,* but with increasing abduction of the arm through positions 1 to 5. *C.* Hands behind head, the movement is backward motion of the elbows, to the floor when supine and to the wall when erect. This motion may be assisted by a therapist and may be resisted. *D.* "Push-ups" from the wall performed in a corner. The exercise starts with hands at waist level; then the hands "climb" until they are fully extended overhead, still apart. The anterior capsule is stretched, as are the pectorals. Rhythm here is necessary. Avoid arching the back and the neck.

freedom to actively move the arm during the application of the pack.

Pain from an acute shoulder tendinitis must be decreased to permit mobilization of the glenohumeral joint. Correspondingly, pain must be decreased to prevent immobilization, disuse, fibrosis, and all the periarticular tissue changes that lead to a "frozen" shoulder.

Analgesics may be employed. The type differs with the experience of the physician and with the previous experience of patient response.

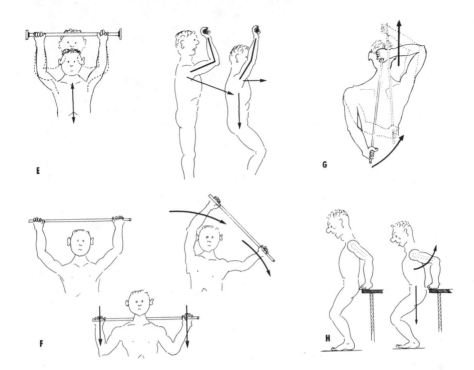

FIGURE 50 (continued). *E.* With a "chinning bar" (between door frames) that is adjustable, begin with the bar at face level and gradually elevate the bar, either by changing the position in the door frame or by doing a deep knee bend. Ultimately the bar should be above and behind the head. *F.* Similar to *E,* except that a "wand" or wooden dowel is held by both hands. This exercise is more active than in *E,* the ultimate object being to place the wand behind the head from a fully extended overhead position. Lateral motion with the arms overhead should attempt movement of arms behind the head. *G.* Wand behind the back. In the illustration the wand is elevated by the right hand to bring the left (involved) arm up behind the back, which stretches the anterior capsule and the external rotators. *H.* Placing hands behind the back upon a table, parallel bars, or sink, and doing deep knee bends.

Opiates, when used sparingly in the first few days, may be necessary. Apprehension, which increases the muscle tension about the inflamed shoulder, must be controlled by sedatives or tranquilizers. Muscle relaxants are numerous on today's pharmaceutical market and all have their advocates. It is a safe assumption presently that there is *no one* effective muscle relaxant and that none is without some sedative effect.

Nonsteroidal anti-inflammatory drugs have great value during the acute phase of tendinitis. They all have potential side effects that should be known to the prescriber and guarded against. Usually daily doses for 5 days are effective. Occasionally several "courses" of these

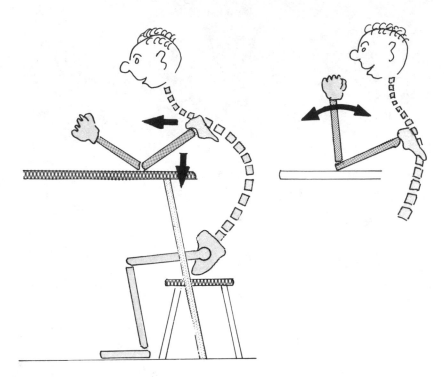

FIGURE 51. Home exercise to increase shoulder range of motion. Seated with arm supported upon table, the patient moves forward and downward to increase range of arm toward elevation. The forearm, bent at right angles, internally and externally rotates, thus further increasing range. A weight can be held in the hand.

drugs are needed. Contraindications to the use of these nonsteroidal anti-inflammatory drugs are well documented in the literature and by the pharmaceutical houses.

Oral steroids may occasionally be indicated and valuable. Large doses for brief periods of time are often of greater value than smaller doses for longer periods. The indications are those of severe symptoms and findings. The contraindications are those of using steroids for any reason.

The use of steroids by injection combined with a local anesthetic agent is very effective. Injection during the first days of an acute attack is usually not indicated. The injection of an anesthetic agent may relieve the acute pain, but the introduction of steroids at this stage is questionable when noninvasive therapy most often is effective.

The rationale of local injection merits discussion. Insofar as the pain-causing tissue is an inflamed, swollen tendon, already weakened and degenerated, further trauma must be avoided. The further trauma alluded to is that caused by the puncture of a needle, introduction of a

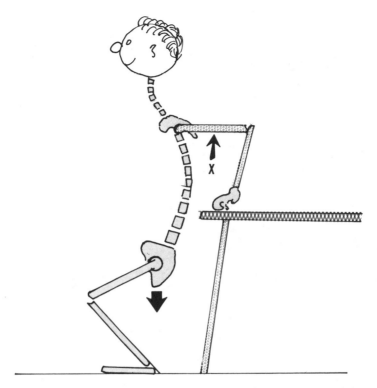

FIGURE 52. Exercise to stretch anterior capsule and increase posterior flexion. The patient places both hands on a table behind the back and performs gentle deep knee bends. This elevates arms (*small arrow*) and increases posterior flexor range of motion.

foreign substance, at best locally irritating, and the introduction of further fluid into a confined area already containing excessive fluid.

The introduction of Novocain is for its anesthetic effect, and cortisone, for its analgesic and anti-inflammatory effect. The amount of fluid is that which is sufficient to separate the inflamed tissues and decrease the formation of adhesions. If the tendon sheath or the tendon is entered, the enclosed debris, acting as a "bulging" sterile abscess within the sheath, may be decompressed. If the bursa is entered, the needle may decompress the inflamed contents of the bursa. All the effects of needle insertion, properly done, are beneficial in that the insertion instills anesthetic and anti-inflammatory solution in an inflamed area and tends to decompress by incising a bulging, fluid mass.

The technique of injection varies with the clinician. The author prefers to use the anterior approach (Fig. 48). Anterior palpation of the shoulder can easily reveal the overhanging acromial process below which is a horizontal sulcus, below which the head of the humerus

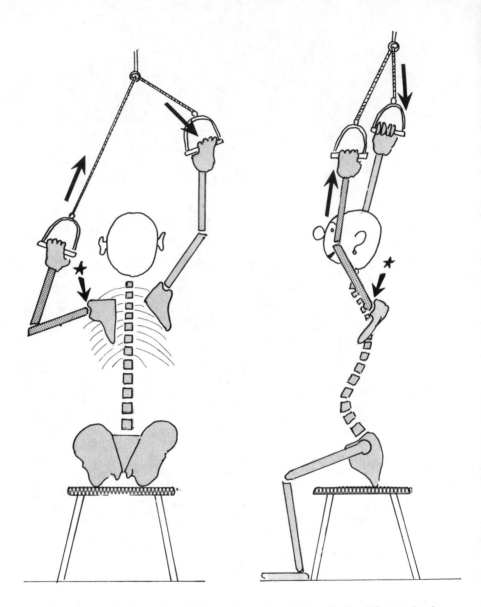

FIGURE 53. Overhead exercise. With a pulley placed above the head the involved arm is passively elevated by the normal arm. By having the pulley slightly behind the head, the arm gets further range of motion to overcome one of the subtle signs of limitation.

and the bicipital grooves can usually be felt. Palpation is done with the arm hanging at the side in a neutral position of rotation. A 2-inch, 24-gauge needle, attached to a 5 cc syringe, filled with 1 cc of 1 percent procaine and 1 cc of injectable steroid (25 mg equivalent of in-

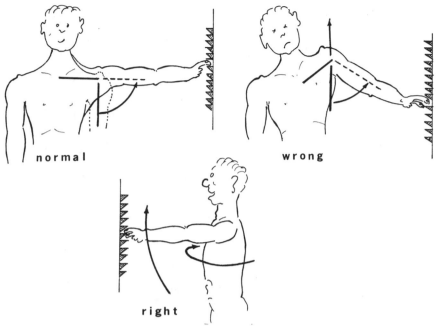

FIGURE 54. Correct and incorrect use of "wall climbing" exercise. The wall climbing exercise frequently is done improperly. The normal arm climbs with normal scapulohumeral rhythm. When there is a pericapsulitis, the wall climb in abduction is done with "shrugging" of the scapula and accomplishes nothing. The wall climb should be started facing the wall and gradually turning the body until the patient is at a right angle to the wall.

jectable steroid) under sterile technique, is inserted anteriorly at a site just above the greater humeral tuberosity (above and lateral to the biceps sulcus) and under the acromion. The needle goes straight back and slightly upward in an attempt to go under the acromium. It is then partially withdrawn and reinserted medially, to follow the supraspinatus tendon. A third reinsertion from partial withdrawal is slightly outward under the tip of the overhanging process. This should infiltrate the subdeltoid bursa if it is at all distended.

The site of needle insertion should be carefully palpated by the finger. The acromial process is easily identified. The biceps groove may need internal and external rotation of the humerus to verify the groove moving under the palpating finger. Downward traction upon the arm may "open" the joint slightly as a few degrees of backward abduction will outline more clearly the protruding humeral tuberosity.

After entering the skin and going through the deltoid muscle, the clinician must exert care to prevent "hitting" bone and injecting into

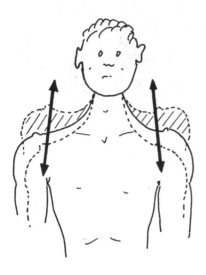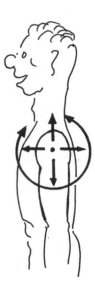

FIGURE 55. Scapular mobility exercises. Previous exercise mobilizes the glenohumeral as well as the scapulothoracic articulations. Motion here is elevation, forward and backward motion, then circumduction of the shoulder girdle. Motion here also increases sternoclavicular and acromioclavicular range of motion.

the periosteum, which will inevitably give "after-injection" pain, often as painful as the condition for which the injection is given. Attempt at aspiration is done to avoid injection into a blood vessel, but rarely is bursal fluid aspirated. Return of joint or bursal fluid should not be the criterion for injecting the mixture of Novocain and injectable steroid.

Aspiration and irrigation of calcific deposits is not advocated by the author and will not be described. This technique is well documented in the literature.[26] Radiotherapy is advocated by some early in acute bursitis.[27] The consensus appears to indicate more favorable results from radiation therapy in the acute cases rather than in the chronic (acute being cases within 10 days of onset of pain, and chronic, after 10 days), and in cases where diagnostic x-rays reveal fine-appearing calcification rather than dense calcifications. In the author's opinion, results from radiation therapy have been disappointing.

To relieve pain about the glenohumeral joint and institute early active motion, a suprascapular nerve block is extremely effective and is relatively simple to perform. The nerve location is shown in Figure 49. The patient is seated with arms at his side. The spine of the scapula is palpated and marked at its vertebral end and its acromial end with a line connecting the two points. This line is bisected and the outer half again bisected. Approximately 1.5 cm above the supe-

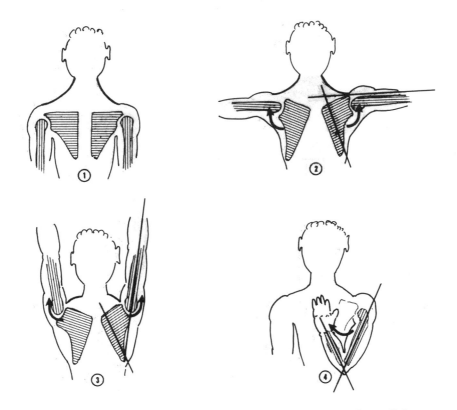

FIGURE 56. Normal scapulohumeral motions: (1) normal stance with parallel symmetric shoulder girdles; (2) symmetric abduction with equal proportional glenohumeral abduction and scapular rotation; (3) symmetric full overhead arm elevation; (4) posterior arm flexion and internal rotation.

rior border of the spine at this point a Novocain wheal is made, and the needle is inserted.

A 24-gauge 2-inch needle is used, connected to a 10 cc syringe containing 1 percent Novocain and 25 mg injectable steroid (hydrocortisone). The needle is advanced slowly until bone is hit. If the nerve is contacted, paresthesia radiating to the shoulder will be elicited. If bone is hit, the needle is withdrawn half the distance and reinserted laterally and medially until paresthesia is elicited. Once the nerve is located, 5 cc of the solution is injected. A complete block should alleviate the pain of the shoulder and produce weakness of arm abduction and external rotation (paresis of the supraspinatus and infraspinatus muscle).

The foregoing technique is aimed at a complete, though transient, nerve block. Since the possibility exists of an overlying vascular bundle, over or behind the notch, rather than to "hit" the nerve directly,

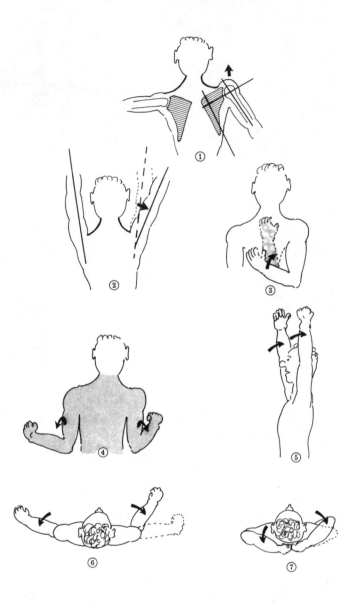

FIGURE 57. Subtle signs of shoulder limitation: (1) shrugging with excessive scapular rotation and limited glenohumeral abduction; (2) limited right arm overhead elevation (arm away from head and ear); (3) limited posterior flexion and internal rotation (hand fails to reach normal interscapular distance of reach); (4) limited external rotation of right arm, done with flexed elbow; (5) overhead elevation of right arm limited in posterior direction as compared with normal, viewed from side; (6) external rotation as viewed from above; (7) with hands behind head, failure of right arm to fully extend posteriorly.

66

the solution is placed under the supraspinatus muscle against the face of the scapular supraspinatus fossa, and allowed to seep along this plane to the nerve. The result is slowed but as effective.[28]

As the acute episode subsides, full recovery must be achieved and recurrence prevented if possible. The "stiff" shoulder and its complications must be prevented. This is possible primarily by *active exercise*. There are advocates of both active exercise and of passive exercise, the latter being equated with *manipulation* as a treatment modality. Both aspects of treatment are efficacious and merit consideration in the treatment armamentarium of the painful stiff shoulder. In summary, the object of treatment is to accomplish full range of pain-free motion of the entire shoulder girdle throughout its range.

Pain noted in abduction of the arm has been attributed to mechanical impingement of the cuff tendons and their contiguous tissues between the humerus and the coracoacromial ligament. Corrective external rotation of the humerus during abduction must occur to move the greater tuberosity posteriorly and thus clear the acromion during abduction. External rotation is thus the key movement in a full-range, pain-free shoulder action. Maintaining or regaining free external rotation is the prime purpose of the postacute phase of treatment.

Elevation of the arm in the sagittal plane is possible with much less probability of impingement which constitutes the first phase of exercise, already discussed under pendular exercise. Since the humeral head must "depress" at the glenohumeral joint to permit abduction, this movement is facilitated by the traction aspect of the pendular exercise. Motion, considered by some to be "involuntary" motion,[29] may require passive (assistive), even forceful, assistance by a therapist or doctor. This will be discussed later.

External rotator exercises may accompany the pendular exercise or follow shortly thereafter. Only the most effective and the simplest exercises will be discussed; they will be described in the legends under the drawings, rather than in the text.

Exercises are classified as (1) *passive* (assistive), in which motion of a joint is performed for the patient; (2) *active*, in which the effort is solely that of the patient; (3) *active assisted*, in which there is a combination of the two; and (4) *active resistive*, where the active effort of the patient is resisted mechanically by equipment or resisted manually by a therapist. All the exercises illustrated (Fig. 50) can be modified into any of these categories.[29]

Individual exercises are shown in Figures 51 through 55. These illustrations can be given to patients for implementation in their home exercise program.

Passive and active unresisted exercises are essentially intended to increase range of motion. Resistance is applied to increase muscular

67

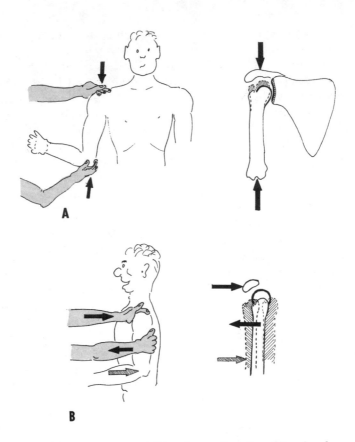

FIGURE 58. Manipulation treatment of "involuntary" motion of the glenohumeral joint. A. Elevation of the head of the humerus against the glenoid fossa. Pressure along the shaft of the humerus, with the other hand preventing elevation of the scapula, causes the humerus to elevate, thus stretching the superior capsule. B. Anterior and posterior motion of the head of the humerus against the glenoid. Three points of contact must be applied. One hand mobilizes the humerus while the other hand "fixes" the scapula. The elbow or forearm is fixed by the therapist's body or elbow.

strength and endurance. Active assistive exercises that involve a second party may vary from forced motion to manipulation.

Exercises should be performed smoothly and with concentration. The patient must understand the purpose of the exercises so that his effort is specific and he avoids substitution of movement. Some sensation, even to the point of discomfort, is bound to occur, but it should never be violent, nor should it leave residual pain and increased disability. A patient who fails to feel some sensation of "stretch," however, is bound not to improve, or at least will reach a plateau of improvement that is never surpassed. Exercises must be done repeatedly, frequently, and correctly. To paraphrase Watson-Jones,

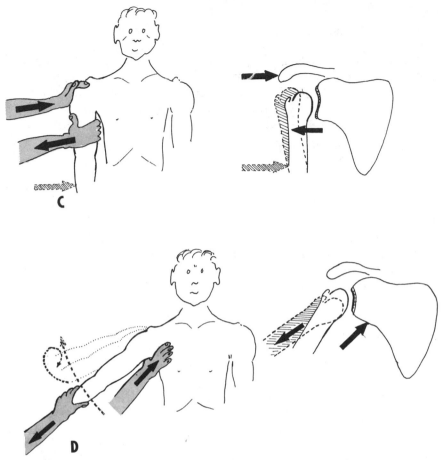

FIGURE 58 (continued). *C*. Lateral motion of the head of the humerus away (in separation) from the glenoid. One hand of the therapist pulls at a right angle to the shaft of the humerus while the scapula and the elbow are "fixed." *D*. Traction to separate the head of the humerus from the glenoid while abducting and gradually externally rotating the arm. Counterresistance (fixation) is applied against the axillary border of the scapula.

"Successful treatment of the stiff shoulder is best summarized in two words, *active exercise.*"[30]

Tolerance of pain or even of discomfort is a human variable and must be considered in the decision of prescription of exercise. In passive people, exercise may be necessary longer than in energetic, well-motivated patients. The combination of disuse and prolonged immobilization in a person with a *periarthritic personality*[31] will frequently lead to a *frozen shoulder.*

A certain number of patients will not improve or will fail to improve past a certain plateau despite intensive adequate treatment. In a portion of these patients the shoulder range of motion remains grossly and visibly limited. Pain persists during the achieved range of motion but most often when further range is attempted.

There are patients, however, who feel they have gained full range of motion and the examiner may, on cursory examination also feel they have regained full range of motion. Pain persists. Often these patients retain limitation that is barely perceptible. They exhibit the *subtle signs* of shoulder pericapsulitis or peritendinitis. *These subtle signs must be sought for in every patient who has gained increased range of motion yet continues to have pain* (Figs. 56 and 57).

These subtle signs include the following:

1. In overhead elevation of the arms the involved arm fails to reach the ear as does the normal arm.
2. In overhead elevation the involved arm does not go as far posteriorly (behind the head) as does the normal arm.
3. With arms at the side external rotation of the involved arm does not rotate outwardly as far as does the normal.
4. In reaching behind the back and attempting to touch the thoracic spine between the shoulder blades the involved arm does not reach the same point as does the normal arm.

Upon finding these *subtle signs* in a symptomatic patient, exercises performed by the patient without assistance will no longer be effective. Assistive exercises now are indicated. Mobilization, manipulation, and active assistive exercises of the rhythmic stabilization type are of value.

The rationale of manipulation is that certain *involuntary* movements of the shoulder girdle can be accomplished through their range of motion only by assistance and force. These movements must be free before active motion is possible. The indications for manipulation must be specific and the techniques of manipulation concise and prudent. Careful clinical examination must be supplemented by recent x-ray studies. In periarticular lesions, manipulation treatment has rationale, whereas articular lesions frequently contraindicate it.[32]

The involuntary movement[33] may be summarized as (1) movement of the humeral head upward upon the glenoid fossa up under the coracoacromial hood; (2) forward movement of the head of the humerus upon the glenoid; (3) backward movement of the humeral head upon the fossa; (4) downward motion of the humerus upon the glenoid; and (5) combination of the above motions. All these motions are apparently aimed at stretching the glenohumeral capsule and releasing adhesions.

Manipulation technique cannot be fully discussed in this text, but skill, based on training, close supervision by a trained person, and

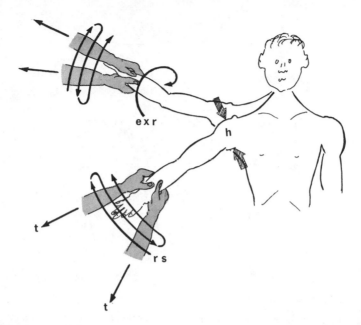

FIGURE 59. Rhythmic stabilization manipulation of the glenohumeral joint. While the patient applies isometric contraction of the glenohumeral joint to "prevent motion," the therapist attempts to move the arm in abduction external rotation, then reverses to adduction internal rotation. Traction (t) is constantly applied. Motion by the therapist is smooth and gradually increasing then decreasing in force and amplitude, with the patient resisting it with equal force. After one cycle at a specific range of abduction, the arm is passively abducted and externally rotated to a further point, and the cycle is repeated.

sound fundamental knowledge of anatomy must precede its application (Fig. 58). Insofar as leverage is a component of the force applied, it behooves the manipulator to use the utmost gentleness and care. *Extreme force is never necessary*,[34] and *abrupt movements must be avoided*.

Manipulation may be done with or without anesthesia. There are advocates of both schools of thought, and there are ardent critics who condemn manipulation under anesthesia as both dangerous and futile.[35] It behooves the physician caring for shoulder problems to be informed of the pros and cons, the indications and contraindications, and the techniques. Judgment regarding their use then can follow the individual's choice.

Prior to manipulation or immediately after the treatment, the subdeltoid bursal area should receive an injection of an anti-inflammatory steroid, an anesthetic agent, and hyaluronidase.[36,37] The steroid in the injected solution allays post-manipulation pain and inflammation, thus minimizing fibroplasia and adhesions.

71

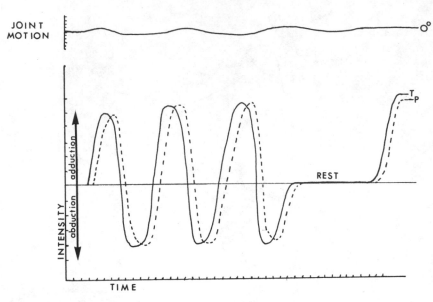

FIGURE 60. Schematic graph of rhythmic stabilization. The solid line (T) indicates the increment of force applied to the shoulder by the therapist in alternating abduction then adduction, immediately followed by opposing force from patient (P) to prevent joint motion (0°).

The increase of motion and decrease of pain permit immediate post-manipulation exercises which are imperative. Active, passive, and active assisted exercises to maintain the gained range of motion and to increase further range must be instituted, supervised, and continued.

Intra-articular injection of an anesthetic agent combined with a steroid, as will be discussed as "infiltration brisement" in Chapter 4 (see also Fig. 63), is of great value to decrease pain and increase mobility utilizing manipulative techniques. The performance of an arthrogram (for diagnosis or for therapy) may be necessary to ascertain that the injected material is *in* the joint space. Through this arthrogram needle a solution of an anesthetic agent (10 cc of 5.0 percent Novocain, lidocaine, or Marcaine) and a steroid are injected into the capsule.

This injection decreases the pain during and after the manipulation and increases the range of motion. This results in better patient cooperation to exercise. This injection can also precede and enhance the benefit of mobilization or "rhythmic stabilization," as it does not decrease voluntary motion.

The author has used effectively a technique of rhythmic stabilization, one that combines active exercises with prudent, controlled manipulation (Fig. 59).[38] The arm, held firmly and with traction, applied manually along the shaft of the humerus, is passively moved in all

72

quadrants of glenohumeral movement. Each movement, foretold by the therapist, is resisted by the patient, causing an isometric contraction of the periarticular muscles but no significant active movement of the joint. After momentary isometric resistance to movement in one direction, the therapist attempts movement in the opposite direction, which the patient immediately resists (Fig. 60).

The back-and-forth passive movement, resisted by an equal force from the patient and done rhythmically, loosens the joint, causes muscular contractions that improve strength and endurance, and improves local blood supply. After a series of alternating contraction-relaxation motions, the arm is *passively* brought to a further point of increased range of motion, and the rhythmic stabilization is done at this newly gained range.

The constant application of traction upon the arm increases the *involuntary* range of motion. The fulcrum created by the position of the therapist and the alternating effort of the patient mobilizes the glenohumeral joint in all the other *involuntary* motions. The patient's active participation allays much of his fear of *"forceful, painful stretch by the therapist."* The need for anesthesia and the encouragement of the postmanipulation effort are therefore minimized.

CHAPTER 3

Cuff Tear

Rupture of the rotator cuff is much more frequent than was previously suspected. Originally, this diagnosis was considered only in people engaged in strenuous occupations who sustained violent trauma, usually a fall. At autopsy tears are frequently noted in people in their early forties who had no previous shoulder complaints.

A minor stress can easily cause a partial or complete tear to a tissue already weakened by degenerative changes. The tissues that tear are enclosed in a small, compact area between the overhanging coracoacromial arch and the gliding humeral head. These tissues are exposed to daily postural, vocational, and traumatic stresses; and in later years, due to a diminishing blood supply, they become more friable.

Nearly all cuff tears occur in the anterior portion of the cuff and are marginal (i.e., close to the point of attachment). Central tears can occur as a linear tear between the tuberosity and the musculotendinous junction, or they can exist along the bicipital groove. Tears can be partial or complete in varying degrees.

DIAGNOSIS

A history of cuff tear occurs most often in men 40 to 50 years of age engaged in hard manual work or experiencing unusual motion, as in recreational sailing. The incidence of "tearing" usually follows a relatively minor injury. The insult may be a fall on the outstretched arm, causing a tear from the arm being "thrown" forward to protect against the fall or the impact against the arm forcing the head of the humerus to penetrate the anterior superior aspect of the cuff. Abduction of the arm without the proper rotatory mechanism can impinge the cuff against the coracoacromial arch and cause a tear. Tears can be iatrogenic from forceful manipulation tearing an already degenerated cuff. Overhead movements of the arm, such as in plastering, painting

74

ceilings, or closing overhead garage doors, may be the tearing stress; but frequently no specific history of trauma or unusual stress can be elicited.

The history is usually of an acute, severe pain described as a "tearing" pain followed by a 6- to 12-hour pain-free interval. This pain-free interval is followed by a gradual return of pain of increasing severity, lasting 4 to 7 days.

Incomplete cuff tears clinically resemble the signs and symptoms of supraspinatius tendonitis. The pathologic reason for this is that the torn fibers retract and "bunch" up, causing an enlargement similar to that of the tendonitis (Fig. 61). Because there are still some intact fibers of the supraspinatus muscle that can assist in abduction and place the humerus in a position to allow the deltoid to act, abduction of the arm is possible, albeit with (1) some pain, (2) some limitation, and (3) an occasional "catch" during the process of abduction. The scapulocostal rhythmn is not impaired.

Resisting abduction and external rotation may produce pain that unresisted movement will not elicit, but this is not diagnostic. Tenderness over the site of the tear is prevalent, and, since the tear occurs most frequently in the supraspinatus portion of the cuff, the tenderness is palpated over the greater tuberosity (see Fig. 44). Occasionally, in very thin persons, a rent in the tendon can be palpated. Diagnosis of an incomplete tear may be made on clinical manifestations, but arthrography may be needed for confirmation.

In a *complete tear* the patient is unable to initiate abduction. The loss of active abduction is caused by the failure of the cuff (especially the supraspinatus) to initiate humerus abduction that places the deltoid into a functional position. Pain may be severe and be considered to be the cause of limited abduction. Even passive abduction may be limited due to pain and confuse the examiner. Early recognition is therefore often difficult.

Injecting an anesthetic agent into the suprahumeral area (see Fig. 48) can remove the pain and relieve the reflex spasm that immobilizes the glenohumeral movement. With relief of pain and spasm clearer diagnostic findings verify the tear. No active abduction is now evident. The patient merely "shrugs" due to scapular motion, but there is no glenohumeral motion (Fig. 62).[39]

The deltoid muscle contracts in spite of the absence of resultant arm abduction, indicating that the axillary nerve is intact and that failure to abduct is not due to nerve damage. If the arm is passively abducted by the examiner, placing the humerus in slight abduction, the arm can be held abducted. By passively placing the arm in abduction, the deltoid now can function as the major abductor.

Because the cuff is not functioning, the head of the humerus is not

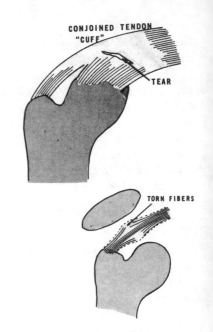

FIGURE 61. Cuff-tear. *Above*: Site and direction of partial cuff tear. *Below*: Retraction of torn cuff fibers forms a thickening of the cuff, thus resembling the thickening of tendinitis.

firmly seated into the glenoid fossa, and thus the glenohumeral joint is not stable. Any downward pressure upon the abducted arm causes it to "drop." The inability of the patient to actively abduct the arm, to actively hold the arm in the abducted position upon the arm being passively placed in abduction and the "drop arm test" upon exerting downward pressure upon the abducted arm, is diagnostic of a complete cuff tear. Arthrography will confirm the presence of a tear and verify whether the tear is complete or incomplete.

Paresis of the deltoid muscle, due to a peripheral nerve injury to the axillary nerve (C_5, C_6) must always be kept in mind when abduction weakness of the deltoid results after an injury.[40]

ARTHROGRAPHY

Contrast dye study of the glenohumeral joint is a safe and simple test that has conclusive value in determining the presence and completeness of a cuff tear. Normally there is no communication of the articular cavity with the subdeltoid bursa. *Communication of the bursa with the articular cavity is abnormal and indicates pathologic rupture* (Fig. 62). The subscapular bursa normally communicates with the joint cavity and is considered a prolongation of the synovial capsule. The subcoracoid bursa is considered by most observers to communicate as well.

The preferred technique of dye injection is by the posterior ap-

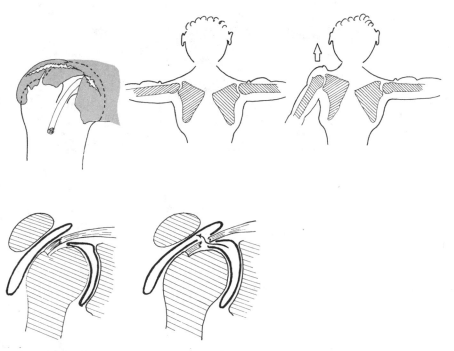

FIGURE 62. Cuff tear. The upper left diagram indicates the usual site of the tear, either partial or complete. The center posterior view of the patient abducting the arm indicates normal or even adequate scapulohumeral movement with a large but incomplete tear. The right view shows the complete tear. The lower diagrams show (*right*) the communication between the shoulder joint in a complete tear, and (*left*) the lack of communication in a partial tear or degenerated tendon.

proach. The posterior approach does not confuse the test if there is leakage, whereas in the anterior approach leakage can mar the final picture (Fig. 63). The site of insertion is a point 1 inch below and 1 inch medial to the angle of the spine of the scapula. A 21-gauge needle attached to a 20 cc syringe is used, filled with Diodrast dye. After 3 or 4 cc of dye is injected, the site of injection is fluoroscopically viewed. If it is considered to be in the joint, an additional 10 to 15 cc is injected.[41,42]

In an intact joint space, having no communication with the subdeltoid bursa, a *reflux* action occurs. The procaine injected backs into the syringe as the plunger pressure is released. No reflux occurs in the presence of a cuff tear because no intracapsular pressure is built up. Approximately 20 cc of dye solution is used, and x-rays are taken with the shoulder in internal and external rotation, as well as an axial view. The dye disappears within several hours with no untoward effects.

The normal arthrogram is depicted in Figure 64. The dye balloons

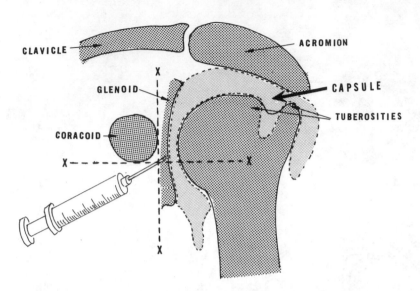

FIGURE 63. Injection technique for intra-articular arthrogram and brisement treatment. The injection site is a point just inferior and lateral to the coracoid process in the vector lines (X–X).

out the capsule, filling the subscapular bursa and the biceps pouch. No dye should appear above the superior border of the humeral head or above and around the greater tuberosity. Appearance of dye into the subdeltoid bursa indicates a pathologic connection. Dye in the bursa appears as a clearly defined "cap" above the humeral head. More fluid is also permitted during the injection (as much as 40 to 50 cc).

An incomplete tear will not form a well-defined "cap" superiorly but may form an abnormal irregularity in the otherwise smooth surface of the normal arthrogram at the site of the greater tuberosity.

"Frozen shoulders" will cause abnormal arthrograms, but not dye invasion into the subdeltoid bursa. Rather the dye will reveal a generally constricted, deformed joint space with poor or no filling of the subscapular bursa or the biceps tendon pouch. Adhesive capsulitis is not usually associated with cuff tears unless the tear is caused by "therapeutic manipulations."

TREATMENT

Incomplete Tears

Two schools of thought regarding the nonsurgical treatment of incomplete cuff tears are diametrically opposed. One concept advocates placing the arm in a position that approximates the torn fibers and

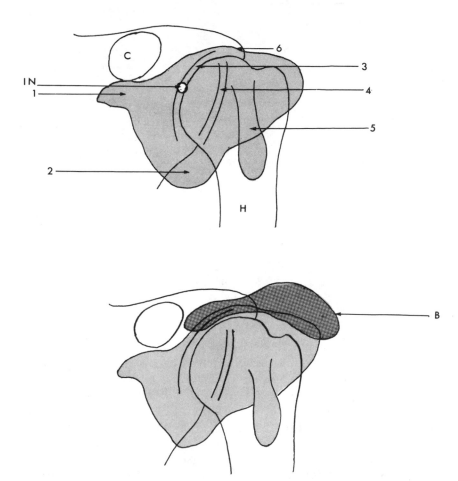

FIGURE 64. Arthrogram. The shaded area on the schematic shoulder joint depicts the normal arthrogram. IN is the anterior site of injection into the glenohumeral joint. 1. The subscapular bursa that normally communicates directly with the shoulder joint and thus fills in a normal gram. 2. As the dye injection distends the capsule, it hangs as a dependent pouch under the joint. 3. The superior medial surface of the humerus. 4. In the arthrogram is a line of lesser density caused by the underlying glenoid labrum. 5. The synovial lining that is the pouch accompanying the biceps tendon sheath in the intertubercular groove a distance of some 2 inches. A rotator cuff tear will permit the dye to extend into the subacromial bursa, superior to the smooth line above the humeral head, above and "around the corner" of the greater tuberosity (B).

eliminating any movement that can elongate the cuff for a period of 8 weeks. The arm is placed in abduction, forward flexion, and external rotation and so held by a plaster spica (Fig. 65).

The rival school of thought advocates immediate *active* motion as soon as pain permits. Exercise is supplemented by frequent injections of Novocain. If abduction from the dependent position is significantly

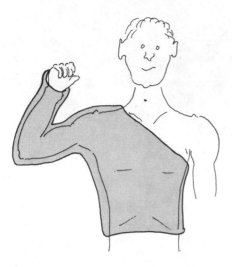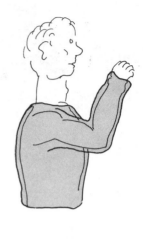

FIGURE 65. Proper spica cast for the torn cuff treatment. The body spica must hold the arm (humerus) abducted, flexed forward, and externally rotated. This is the position of least tension upon the rotator cuff and therefore that of maximum opposition of the torn ends of the cuff.

weak, an abduction splint is applied, and active abduction exercises are started from that level of abduction. The use of the splint, as an assistive device for the exercise, is usually needed for 3 weeks, and the total exercise program results in a pain-free shoulder action within 8 weeks. This active exercise concept, with no immobilization, is especially advocated in the older age group in which immobilization of even brief duration can lead to a "frozen shoulder."

There are advocates of surgical repair of the incomplete cuff tear with brief immobilization then exercise following the repair.[43]

Complete Tears

Surgical repair is indicated immediately upon diagnosing a complete tear. The surgical techniques are beyond the scope of this text but are well documented in the literature.[2,9,35] Postoperative care frequently determines the efficacy of the surgery regardless of the operation chosen. Here, as in the treatment of incomplete tears, the treatment varies from complete immobilization in a plaster spica to suspending the arm in a splint immediately after surgery and beginning gentle passive movement on the following day. Gradually, passive motion, then active assisted motion is begun, with forward flexion preceding abduction. By the fourth week, the arm is gradually lowered but is returned to the splint at night. The arm is held in the splint between exercise periods until the arm can be abducted, unassisted, against gravity. Resistive exercises are judiciously and gradually started.

A supervised, active exercise treatment program offers the best results in both the incomplete and the postoperative complete tears.

CHAPTER 4

Adhesive Capsulitis: The "Frozen Shoulder"

"Frozen shoulder" is a term widely used but poorly understood. The concept has varied meanings, as is evident by the many terms that are used synchronously and the varied pathologic conditions attributed to the clinical picture. The condition has been referred to as adhesive capsulitis, periarthritis, pericapsulitis, obliterative bursitis, "stiff shoulder," the shoulder component of the "shoulder-hand" syndrome, and scapulohumeral periarthritis, among others.

The syndrome of "frozen shoulder" relates to the stiff shoulder in which movement, both active and passive, is restricted and painful at the scapulothoracic joint as well as at the glenohumeral joint, is without demonstrable intrinsic cause, has no osseous ankylosis, responds differently to different forms of treatment, and usually has a self-limited duration with gradual recovery ultimately expected in the majority of cases. A relatively small percentage of cases remain permanently "frozen."

"Frozen shoulder" must be considered a clinical rather than a pathologic entity.[32] Any of the causes of pain felt in the shoulder may initiate a stiff shoulder, but the "frozen shoulder" occurs mostly when the factors of *disuse* coexist in a person with deep-seated tension, anxiety, and passive apathy (the so-called *periarthritic personality*[31]), together with a low pain threshold. The progression of the disability has been diagrammed in Figure 45, and is more specifically keyed to the "frozen shoulder" in Figure 66.

Figure 66 is self-explanatory in its total concept, but many of the stages leading to fibrous reaction are not evident. Pain can cause vasospasm by an intricate connection of sensory nerves, their posterior root ganglia, and the sympathetic nervous system.[44] The idea of vasospasm (and the concurrent tissue ischemia) as an initiator of pain is questionable. Pain (in causalgia) has been attributed to vasospasm, but the sensation of pain was identical regardless of ischemia or hyperemia;

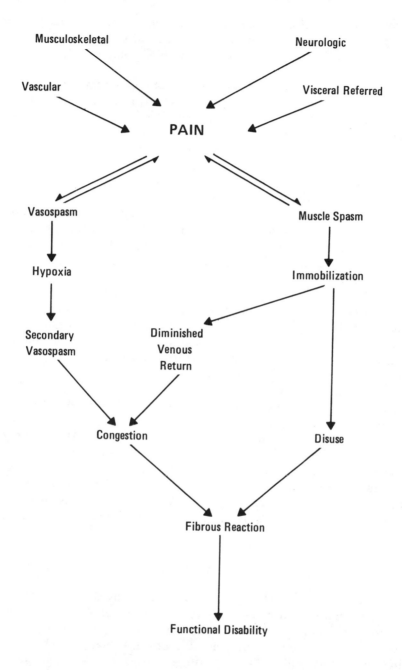

FIGURE 66. Schematic stages toward functional disability in the painful shoulder.

therefore, *pain causes, rather than is caused by, vasospasm.*[45] Studies of vegetative function, such as vasospasm and trophic changes, were not found to differ in "periarthritic patients" compared to normal patients.[46]

Muscle spasm is a protective mechanism to prevent movement that is painful. The passive, apathetic patient who is reluctant to exert effort, or the patient with a low pain threshold who will not tolerate the slightest pain, will "splint" the arm to the side in a dependent position. This immobile dependency will cause venous stasis and secondary congestion, which, combined with vasospastic anoxia, will lead to a protein-rich, edematous exudate and ultimate fibrous reaction.

In the "frozen shoulder" the proliferative inflammatory edema occurs in the region of the *osteofibrous case*[7] about the glenohumeral joint. This case is composed of loose connective tissue on either side of a fascial sheath between the undersurface of the deltoid and the outer surface of the rotator cuff (Fig. 67).[7] This subdeltoid fascia is rich in blood vessels and sympathetic nerve endings.

Irritation to the osteofibrous case of the suprahumeral vault can be from any of the factors cited in Figure 66 and outlined at the opening of Chapter 2. The irritant initiates cellular exudate, vasospasm, and venous congestion. Immobilization and a hyperreactive vasomotor response lead to fibrosis. Fibrosis leads to adhesions occurring between the layers of the osteofibrous case.

This reasonably simple explanation discloses the many pathologic concepts of the *frozen shoulder*: (1) adhesions between layers of the subdeltoid bursa;[1,47] (2) extra-articular and intracapsular adhesions;[2] (3) contracture of the subscapularis and biceps tendon;[48] (4) adherence of the anterior-inferior folds of the joint capsule to each other (Fig. 68) and to the adjacent glenoid and humerus,[49] so-called adhesive capsulitis; (5) obliterative bursitis; and (6) myostatic contracture, the contracted "stiffening" of the girdle muscles.[50] All these concepts fit into the fibrous reaction within the case and follow the mechanism outlined in Figure 66.

DIAGNOSIS

A "frozen shoulder" should be suspected when a painful limitation of the glenohumeral joint becomes less painful but increasingly more limited in motion. The initial limitation caused by reflex spasm is the result of vascular hyperemia, and all motion is guarded. This stage is limited to a period of 7 to 10 days, depending upon treatment, severity of the causative factors, and the patient's response.

After the acute phase some restriction persists, and some pain can result, far exceeding the allowable movement. Pain will result when

FIGURE 67. Periarticular case of the suprahumeral joint. The lining and contained tissues of the suprahumeral joint are graphically depicted as a "case." The superior layer is the undersurface of the deltoid, and the floor is the outer surface of the rotator cuff. Interposed is loose connective tissue (ct) and a strong subdeltoid fascia (f). The fascia is richly endowed with blood vessels and sympathetic nerve endings. Proximally the fascia contains the coracoacromial ligament (not shown) and ends distally in the periosteum of the humerus at the level of the surgical neck.

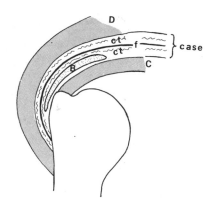

the tissues that remain inflamed are irritated or compressed. In supraspinatus tendinitis abduction remains limited because of the encroachment of the inflamed tendon under the coracoacromial arch. External rotation is limited because of involvement of the subscapularis, and involvement of the infraspinatus and the teres minor causes pain on internal rotation. *Adduction* and forward-backward swing in the sagittal plane (see Fig. 17) should remain free.

As the shoulder becomes "frozen," pain is absent when the arm is immobile. Motion becomes restricted in *all* ranges, including abduction and movement in the sagittal plane. The arm becomes immobile against the chest wall with the arm adducted, internally rotated, and dependent. Any attempt at active or passive motion is increasingly resisted, and stretch pain occurs when forceful movement is attempted. Varying degrees of limitation exist; but the untreated result is total immobility, and no active and no passive motion is permitted. Any motion of the shoulder complex is performed at the scapula, and this with limitation.

TREATMENT

The *optimal treatment of a frozen shoulder is that of prevention.* Once the "frozen shoulder" syndrome is initiated, treatment, and certainly cure, is increasingly more difficult. Although the "frozen shoulder" is considered a self-limited disease process that, given time, will "ultimately recover," complete recovery with no residual limitation and disability is neither assured nor common.

Fibrosis, secondary arthritis, myostatic contracture, osteoporosis, and severe disuse atrophy may be permanent. Only *active* use of the arm and full maintenance of the glenohumeral movement will prevent these changes.

Treatment of the patient with the painful stiff shoulder is a dual

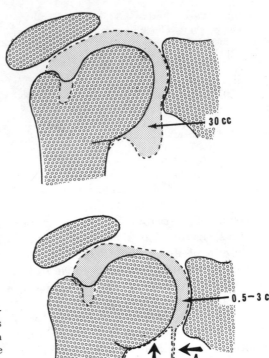

FIGURE 68. Adhesive capsulitis. The normal capsule permits injection of at least 30 cc of air. In adhesive capsulitis, the capsule adheres to itself (A) and to the humeral head (B). This decreases capacity to 0.5 to 3 cc and markedly limits range of motion.

process. Treatment must be directed to the arm locally and must also take into consideration treatment of the whole patient. As has been alluded to, this "frozen" shoulder complication occurs most often in intrinsically tense people; people in a sustained tense situation; patients of a passive, dependent nature; and patients with low pain threshold and a vasomotor liability. Local treatment to the arm that requires active effort, movement painful to a degree, and treatment carried on for an adequately long period must be instituted. The patient must be able and willing to cooperate.

When possible the stressful situation and environment enveloping the patient must be manipulated and reduced. Anxiety not directly related to the arm must be dissipated, and anxiety regarding the arm must be quelled. Knowledge regarding the cause of the painful shoulder must be discussed. The patient must be constantly reassured. Assistance, at first passive, but with a goal of active participation, must be carefully offered. If deemed necessary for a patient so severely disturbed emotionally that adherence to a physical program is difficult, psychotherapy may be necessary as an adjunct to local therapy.

Drugs play a large role in treating the potentially stiff shoulder. Muscle relaxants are employed, but a generally effective muscle relaxant is also usually a tranquilizer and a sedative. The fact that tranquilizers have been so effective in the drug management of the potentially stiff, painful shoulder with release of the "spasm" and limitation has led the author to accept the idea that "tension myositis"—the connotation of "tension" being emotional tension—is a significant component of the stiffening process. Personal experience with a specific drug, be it a tranquilizer or a muscle relaxant, becomes a part of each physician's armamentarium; and with the current increase in the number of varied drugs appearing on the market, no specific drug will be advocated here.

Care must be exercised to avoid causing depression in prescribing drugs that tranquilize or sedate.[51,52] Depression may decrease a patient's willingness and ability to cooperate actively. Depression affects the posture, which furthers the mechanically damaging "droopy shoulder" attitude previously described (see Fig. 39). Depression caused by drugs may result in the patient's discouragement at the expected slow progress and early discontinuance of an otherwise effective treatment.

Pain medications are valuable, but narcotics should be avoided except for very brief periods during the early and severe pain periods. When possible, analgesic compounds, even salicylate compounds, should be utilized if they control the pain.

Drugs of the phenylbutazone series (e.g., Butazolidin) are extremely valuable. They should be used in large doses for brief periods when not specifically contraindicated (e.g., 200 mg t.i.d. for 3 days). Oral steroids fall into the same category and may be spectacular in their effectiveness (e.g., prednisone, 20 mg daily for 5 days). Judicious and knowledgeable use of the drug is obviously necessary.

Local injections of procaine and steroids help when pain is severe and palpable local tenderness localizes the site of injection. Multiple injections of steroid in a diffusely tender shoulder with no localizing "trigger" area or multiple injections that fail to improve the symptoms satisfactorily should be discontinued and a course of antiphlogistic drug or oral steroids substituted.

Nerve blocks are valuable adjunctive therapy to facilitate active exercise. Stellate ganglion block that interrupts the pain fibers traveling along the shoulder sympathetic nerve is advocated by some. Suprascapular nerve block (described in Fig. 49) is an effective and simple measure for relieving shoulder pain.

Manipulation of the shoulder under anesthesia is not advocated and, in fact, is considered by many to be contraindicated.[53] Those who do advocate manipulation consider active exercise to be imperative immediately after the manipulation and for a period thereafter. However, can we expect a patient whose inability or unwillingness to move a painful joint has led to the "freezing" to move the shoulder that has been made excruciatingly more painful by the manipulation? Forceful external rotation can tear the cuff tendons, especially the subscapularis. Fracture of the humerus osteoporotic from disuse is not uncommon. The advocates of manipulation,[7] emphasize that mobilization of the shoulder under anesthesia be done with "a delicate sense of touch" and that, even properly done, it "is useless and gives poor results unless followed by extremely careful after-treatment." Good technique of manipulation can be acquired, but cooperation of the "frozen-shoulder" patient is not easily obtained.

X-ray treatment is of little nonspecific value, as is ultrasound therapy. Surgical intervention should be avoided except where there is an incriminating hard calcific mass or a complete cuff tear.

Although there are many who claim that adhesive capsulitis is self-limited and "in time resolves," there are too many patients who have persistent, albeit painless, "frozen shoulders." A form of treatment has been advocated that is termed *infiltration brisement*[54] (see Fig. 63). Under a general anesthetic a needle is inserted into the capsule. As in the performance of an arthrogram, dye is injected to ascertain that the capsule has been entered. It must be remembered that in adhesive capsulitis the capsule admits very little fluid (perhaps 3 cc). Once in the capsule two 50 cc Luer lock syringes filled with 0.3 percent Xylocaine (or a similar anesthetic agent) and 20 cc triacimilone are fitted to the needle and forcefully injected into the capsule. The pressure exerted upon the syringe plunger is what can be exerted manually.

At a certain point a sudden "give" is felt which indicates rupture of the capsule. The arm can then be passively abducted to full range of motion. Immediately after the injection active physical therapy must be administered.

Passive and active range of motion exercises must be instituted. An abduction splint of plaster or metal and leather can be applied that maintains the arm in abduction and slight external rotation.

Ice applied locally is beneficial. Active exercises done by the patient hourly are valuable. The determination of the patient before brisement is considered must be known to insure active cooperation by the patient following the injection; otherwise the procedure will fail and will often be followed by more pain and as much, if not more, limitation. Active range of motion exercises must be done to insure maintenance of the gained range of motion and further increase in range.

The injected anesthetic agent and the steroid usually decrease pain. Should there be severe pain after the initial brisement, further injections of anesthetic-steroid solution may be administered interarticularly. The tear caused in the capsule apparently heals sufficiently to permit physiologic motion.

Following any form of treatment—brisement, manipulation, intra-articular injection, suprascapular nerve block, or rhythmic stabilization—active exercises must be started and continued faithfully and frequently. Passive exercises may also be needed to insure increased range of motion. *Full range of motion is the goal, as any residual limitation may initiate further pain limitation and another "frozen shoulder."*

Daily exercises are indicated once full range has been gained. Overhead stretching and full external rotation are exercises that should be done repeatedly during the day. To clasp the hands behind the head with elbows back requires the maximum external rotation and abduction.[55] Daily hanging from an overhead chinning bar or reaching for the ceiling or door frame above the head and slightly behind the body is excellent. It has been truly stated that the shoulder joint was designed for arboreal rather than erect biped existence, and that were man swinging from tree to tree rather than standing upright and bending forward at the trunk with arms dangling, the "stiff painful shoulder" would be very rare.[56]

CHAPTER 5

Neurologic Referred Pain

Pain in the shoulder and upper extremity may arise from involvement of the nervous system at a distal point but be felt in the shoulder girdle area. This pain may be traced to involvement of the vertebral column, brachial plexus, or peripheral nerves of the upper extremity. Diagnosis is tantamount to proper treatment.

CERVICAL NERVE ROOT PRESSURE (RADICULITIS)

The most common neurologic source of pain is radiculitis of a cervical nerve root due to cervical spondylosis, or cervical disk herniation. The relationship of the nerve root within the intervertebral foramen is shown in Figure 69. Normally the root is enclosed in a sleeve, and during normal movements of the neck the root is not compressed or irritated. This patency of the foramen is maintained in spite of relative closure of the foramen during the act of neck extension (Fig. 70A and B) and lateral flexion and rotation of the head (Fig. 71).

During normal extension of the neck the cervical vertebrae glide backward on each other, the upper upon the next lower, with approximation of the posterior structures[38] and a physiologic closure of the foramen. Lateral flexion and rotation of the neck and head cause closure of the foramina on the side *toward* which the head rotates and closes on the side *toward* which the neck laterally flexes (Fig. 71). In a normal or well-compensated cervical spine the nerve root is not irritated or compressed.

In cervical diskogenic disease the usual root compression occurs at the interspace between the fifth and sixth or the sixth and seventh cervical vertebrae with compression of the C_6 or C_7 nerve root. Typically the neck is stiff and painful, and paresthesia is claimed down the lateral aspect of the arm and into the fingers. Weakness of the segmental myotome can be elicited. If root pressure is from a herniated

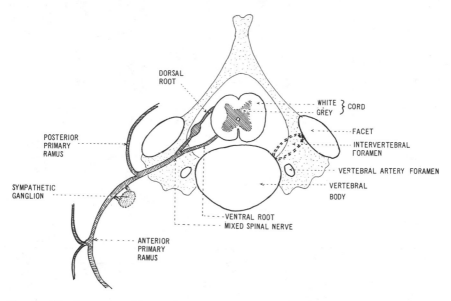

FIGURE 69. Component fibers of a cervical nerve. The relationship of the spinal cord and cervical spinal nerve to the vertebral body, the intervertebral disk, and facet.

cervical disk, flexion of the neck usually causes or aggravates the pain and paresthesia. In the presence of cervical spondylosis (so-called degenerative arthritis),[38] extension of the neck will narrow the intervertebral foramen and impinge the hypertrophied joints of Luschka against the entrapped nerve root (Fig. 70D).

Compression of the C_6 root causes pain and stiffness of the neck, pain and numbness into the thumb and first finger, weakness of the biceps muscle, and depression of the biceps reflex. The referred pain to the shoulder is vague. "Shoulder pain" is more a dull ache in the lateral deltoid region and in the upper interscapular region (Fig. 72).

Compression of the C_7 root causes the numbness and pain to refer to the middle and index fingers with weakness of the triceps muscle and a depressed triceps jerk. The "shoulder" area of referral is also the posterior lateral aspect of the deltoid and the superior medial aspect of the scapula. The C_8 root shoulder area referral is more in the lower trapezius area and over the scapular area (Fig. 72).[57]

Differential diagnosis of the primary shoulder musculoskeletal pain from cervical referred pain should be considered, but once considered, it presents no differential problem. The "shoulder pain" is vague and is reproducible by neck motion, usually forced extension *and* rotation to the side of complaint. Paresthesia of the hand and fingers is claimed, and neurologic deficit of motor weakness and reflex changes are usual. Movement of the shoulder is free and does not

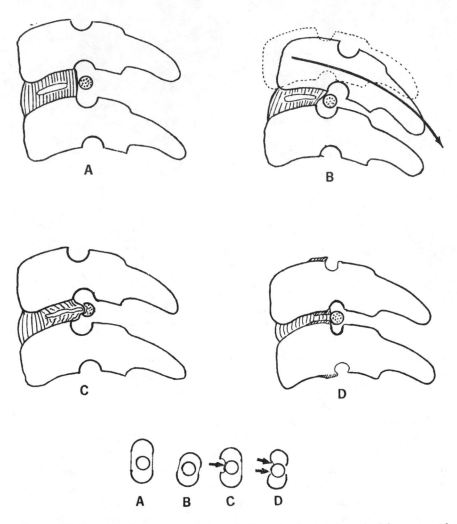

FIGURE 70. Foraminal opening variations. *A*. Normal open intervertebral foramen with neck in neutral position, no rotation and no lateral flexion. *B*. Extension by backward gliding of the upper upon the lower vertebra normally narrows the foramen but does not compress the nerve root. *C*. Compression of the nerve root by herniation of the intervertebral disk. *D*. Distortion of the foramen by osteophytic changes of the joints of Luschka and disk degeneration.

reduplicate the symptoms. The *"shrugging" of the pericapsulitis* and the *scalene spasm of the cervical diskogenic syndrome,* however, may tax the acumen of the examiner.

Diagnosis of cervical diskogenic disease is made principally on the basis of history and physical examination. X-rays of the cervical spine are not diagnostic per se, and even myelography is not conclusive.

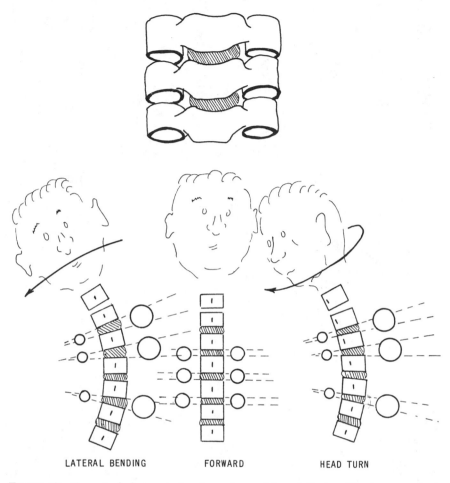

FIGURE 71. Foraminal closure in head rotation and lateral flexion. The intervertebral foramina close on the side toward which the head rotates or bends laterally, and they open on the opposite side.

Response to treatment consisting of traction, collar immobilization, neck exercises, and posture training may be a conclusive factor.

SPINAL CORD TUMOR

Tumors within the spinal canal of the cervical spine may mimic a cervical disk herniation in the early stages, but ultimately there is progression of symptoms and findings. Single nerve root involvement leads to multiple and bilateral roots being involved. Inevitably there is compression of the spinal cord, causing upper motor neuron signs

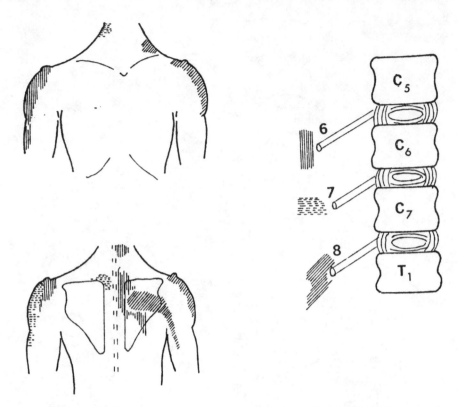

FIGURE 72. Regions of shoulder pain referral from cervical radiculitis. The areas depicted by hatching are the areas of vague "shoulder area" referrals frequently complained of by patients. These are not the cervical root dermatomes which are more specific in C_6, C_7, and C_8 and are referred to the hand, forearm, and fingers. The areas shown in this diagram may be derived from posterior primary rami, or sclerotomes, or they may be areas of myalgic tenderness.

with weakness and incoordination of the legs and bowel-bladder dysfunction.

Diagnosis is suggested by the progressive story and findings, multiple segmental levels, and upper motor neuron involvement. Lumbar puncture revealing abnormal manometrics and elevated protein determinations suggest pantopaque myelography and surgical exploration.

BRACHIAL PLEXUS INVOLVEMENT

The brachial plexus may be the origin of pain felt in the shoulder region; the etiology is conveniently classified into (1) traumatic and (2) mechanical, nontraumatic irritation.

Trauma to the brachial plexus may be caused by penetrating wounds, fracture-dislocation of adjacent bone structures, or traction injuries. Injuries to the brachial plexus from shoulder dislocation and clavicle fracture-dislocation have been discussed under these subjects. Stretch injury to the brachial plexus from distraction between the neck and arm may present a diagnostic problem, since the symptom of severe pain may present minimal objective findings. In this condition the history of traction can be elicited. There is tenderness by deep pressure over the neurovascular bundle and the scalene muscles in the supraclavicular fossa, and pain can be reproduced by placing stretch on the plexus from distraction of the neck and arm.

Objective findings will implicate sensory and motor involvement of many roots—C_5 to T_1—and many require electromyography for verification.

Mechanical nontraumatic brachial plexus compression includes the clinical conditions encompassed in the cervical dorsal outlet syndrome, which includes the cervical rib syndrome, the anterior scalene syndrome, the pectoralis minor syndrome, the costoclavicular syndrome, and the first thoracic rib syndrome. All the symptoms attributed to this syndrome imply compression of the brachial plexus or the subclavian artery, or both, by bony, ligamentous, or muscular obstacles somewhere between the cervical spine and the lower border of the axilla. The most common site is the supraclavicular region in the crowded area containing the first rib, the clavicle, and lower cervical spine with all the tissues contained therein (Fig. 73).

Many of the symptoms originally attributed to the neurovascular compression syndrome, at the thoracic inlet, have recently been attributed to compression irritation of the cervical root at the foraminal level from disk disease, or compression of the median nerve at the wrist. The latter compression results from volar carpal ligament pressure causing "carpal tunnel syndrome" symptoms of numbness, tingling, and weakness, similar to more proximal plexus compression.

SCAPULOCOSTAL SYNDROME

A frequent cause of shoulder pain with localized tenderness and radiation into distal portions of the arm and hand is the scapulocostal syndrome. It is claimed that this syndrome constitutes 90 percent of all cases of cervicobrachial pain.[58]

This syndrome is also called postural fatigue and affects patients during their periods of rest. Gravity upon the scapular components is considered the cause of this syndrome.

As this syndrome also causes symptoms of neurovascular compression in the supraclavicular fossa it is associated with symptoms attri-

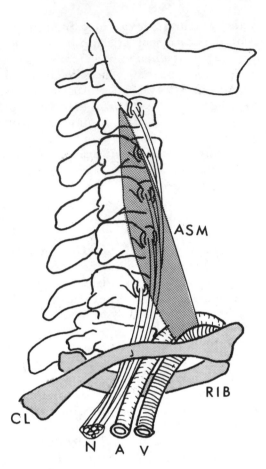

FIGURE 73. Cervical dorsal outlet. Schematic depiction of the course of the brachial plexus subclavian bundle from the cervical spine over the first rib, and under the clavicle (CL) with the relationship to the anterior scalene muscle (ASM). (A = Subclavian artery; N = brachial plexus; V = subclavian vein.)

buted to cervical rib, anterior scalene syndrome, claviculocostal syndrome, and the pectoralis minor syndrome. Each *may* be a specific disease entity, but *all* are related to the single entity of *scapulocostal postural fatigue*. Certainly the kinesiomechanics of this syndrome prevails in all the associated syndromes, and the treatment is similar in all.

The symptoms occur in the patient while at rest in the upright position (sitting or standing). The principal aspect of the syndrome is a downward rotation of the scapulocostal motion of the scapula which rotates the superior-medial aspect of the scapula upward and laterally.

With the downward sagging of the scapula traction upon the levator scapulae muscle occurs, causing this muscle to become irritated and ischemic, and thus go into "spasm." The irritated muscle and the local "trigger" area that develops in the muscle become the clinical symptom and physical finding that are characteristic of the syndrome (Fig. 74).

The following additional symptoms may develop:

1. Hemicranial pain (unilateral headache).
2. Pain in the posterolateral aspect of the neck.
3. Radicular symptoms down the ipsilateral upper extremity that are either vascular or neurologic, or both. The paresthesia may be unilateral or bilateral, and usually is in the ulner nerve distribution.

Many of the symptoms, albeit postural, are related to tension upon the pre- and postvertebral fascia that cause symptoms of myofascilitis with local and referred symptoms. Moreover, due to the anatomic proximity of nerves (brachial plexus) and blood vessels (subclavium), symptoms referable to the neurovascular bundle are explainable.

Anatomy of the Fascia

The prevertebral fascia is a firm membrane lying anteriorly to the prevertebral muscles (longus cervicis, longus capitis, anterior middle and posterior scalenes, and the rectus capitis muscles). It is attached to the base of the skull just anterior to the capitis muscles and descends downward and laterally to ultimately blend with the fascia of the trapezius muscle. In its course it covers the scalene muscles and also binds down the subclavian artery and the three trunks of the brachial plexus (Fig. 75).

The prevertebral fascia crosses (medially) to the transverse processes of the cervical vertebrae and covers all the cervical nerve roots. The fascia *does not* ensheath the subclavian or axillary *veins* and therefore does not cause venous congestion. The fascia is firmly adherent to the anterior aspects of the cervical vertebrae and to the clavicle.

In the posture causing the scapulocostal syndrome symptoms the depressed scapula places strain upon the fascia as well as the scapular musculature. This fascial tension, by causing pressure or traction upon the greater occipital nerve (via the deep cervical fascia), may well account for the associated hemicranial pain.

Traction upon the muscles of the scapula, the trapezius, and the

97

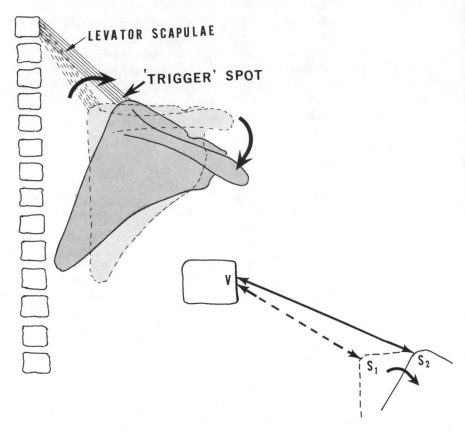

FIGURE 74. Levator scapulae "trigger" zone in postural fatigue syndrome. With lateral downward rotation of the scapula (*curved arrows*) the superior medial angle of the scapula moves the insertion of the levator scapulae muscle (V-S_1 to V-S_2). The muscle under this traction becomes ischemic, inflamed, and thus tender and painful at the "trigger" site.

levator scapulae causes pain in these muscles. Deep tenderness and possibly nodules in these muscles are responsible for the symptoms of myofasciitis in this region.[58]

Obliteration of the radial pulse, as noted in the Adson maneuver (see below), can be attributed to tension of the cervical fascia on rotation of the head and neck. Traction upon the lower trunk of the brachial plexus may well cause the pain and numbness in the ulnar distribution of the hand which is so common in this syndrome.

Fibromyositis has generally become recognized as a specific pathology that persists after trauma, manifested clinically by painful muscles, nodules, spasm, and stiffness of joint motion, both actively and passively.[59,60] This condition has been designated as fibrositis,

98

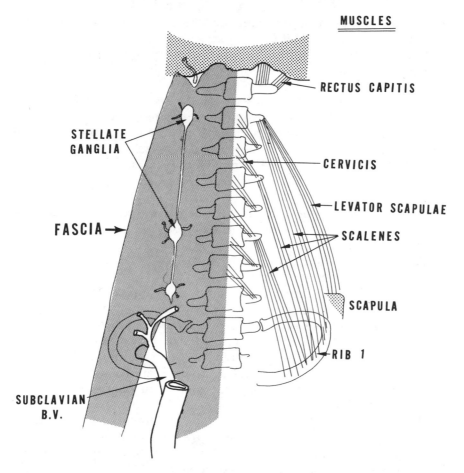

MUSCLES

RECTUS CAPITIS

STELLATE
GANGLIA

CERVICIS

LEVATOR SCAPULAE

FASCIA →

SCALENES

SCAPULA

RIB 1

SUBCLAVIAN
B.V.

FIGURE 75. Anterior view of prevertebral fascia and muscles. The fascia is a firm membrane in front of the prevertebral neck muscles. It binds these muscles to the subclavian artery and three trunks of the brachial plexus. All the cervical nerve roots are beneath the fascia. The fascia is attached to the anterior margin of the cervical vertebral bodies and to the clavicle. The cervical sympathetic trunk lies in front of the fascia.

myofasciitis, myofibrositis, interstitial myofasciitis, and psychogenic rheumatism, among many other descriptions.

The actual existence of fibromyositis has been questioned as there are no confirmatory laboratory findings. Patients do not have fever, leukocytosis, increased sedimentation rate, or alteration of serum enzyme levels.[61] Electromyographic abnormalities have been claimed, but none are consistently and universally accepted.[62] On the assumption that nodules are inflammatory ("trigger points"), steroids have also been injected as well as anesthetic agents. The inflammatory nature of the nodules has been questioned, as many beneficial results have been achieved by the injection of sterile saline or merely dry needling of the painful site.[63]

The symptoms of hemicranial pain (headache) are attributed to one or more of the following:

1. Pressure upon the greater occipital nerve exerted by the deep cervical fascia (in the posterior triangle of the neck).
2. Tension upon the periosteum of the cranium at the attachment of the trapezium or the levator scapulae muscles (traction).
3. Referred pain of cervical origin from increased lordosis causing nerve root entrapment at the intervertebral foramen.[64]

Due to thoracic kyphosis of the "fatigue posture" the fourth and fifth thoracic nerves can be irritated, causing referred pain at the inferior angle of the scapula.

The clinical diagnosis is made by:

1. Observation of the posture: dorsal "round back" kyphosis, with increased compensatory cervical lordosis and a forward head posture. The presence of sagging shoulders. Histories obtained of the causative factor(s) contributing to this posture also confirm in making the diagnosis and in outlining the proper treatment.
2. Elicitation of the "trigger areas" in the scapular antigravity muscles. This may require a careful, meticulous search for the "trigger point" or the referred zone with digital pressure.
3. Elicitation of the neurovascular symptoms and findings by means of the tests described in subsequent sections of this chapter, including the Adson sign, the pectoralis minor test, scalene signs, and claviculocostal signs.[65-67]

Treatment

Treatment is basically correction of the faulty posture with amelioration or correction of the causative factors, including depression, work habits, sitting or standing posture, and self-image.

Improvement of the hypotonic shoulder girdle muscles is also indicated (Figs. 76 and 77). Moist heat application to the neck and shoulders for a period of 20 to 30 minutes. Massage of the deep, painful, indurated muscles is valuable.

Injection of an anesthetic agent into the "trigger" tender area with or without a steroid affords relief. Ethyl chloride or vasocoolant spray to the painful tender muscle, followed by stretching of that specific muscle, also has been advocated.[68-70] Cervical traction and sleeping with a cervical pillow complements the therapeutic regime.

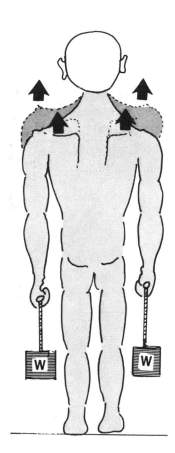

FIGURE 76. Standing scapular elevation exercises. With proper posture (tilted pelvis and flattened cervical lordosis) both arms are rhythmically elevated, held, and slowly lowered. Increasing weights are used. Elbows must be fully extended.

CERVICAL RIB

In the human, only the thoracic spine has fully developed ribs, but occasionally in the cervical spine the transverse process may be overdeveloped or have a supernumerary rib. This is usually bilateral, predominantly in women, and occurs in less than 1 percent of the population. It seldom gives rise to symptoms.

Symptoms attributable to cervical ribs are vascular or neurologic, or both. The vascular signs are rarely severe and mainfest themselves by numbness and tingling of the fingertips. Neurologic symptoms include pain, hypesthesia, hyperesthesia, or paresthesia. Weakness may be present. The neurologic symptoms seen result predominantly from involvement of the eighth cervical and first thoracic nerves, with pain and numbness of the ulnar border of the hand and the last two phalanges of the ring and little fingers, and weakness of the small muscles of the hand. It is difficult to visualize compression of the firm nerve trunk without simultaneous compression of the blood vessels.

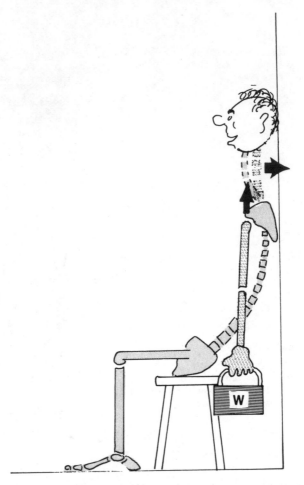

FIGURE 77. Posture-scapular elevation exercises. Patient is seated with back to wall, his head and neck pressed against the wall, which decreases the cervical lordosis. With arms full extended and dependent, weights are lifted in a shrugging motion. Weights vary from 5 to 30 pounds.

Therefore, without vascular changes, a diagnosis of cervical rib compression should be made cautiously.[71]

Treatment should be an intensive, prolonged, conservative regimen of exercises to (1) improve posture, and (2) improve muscle tone of the shoulder girdle. Even a mechanical brace assist to shoulder elevation may be necessary. Surgery, either to resect a cervical rib or to section the scalene muscle, should be the last resort, unless organic impairment of the subclavician artery is suspected. A "bruit" associated with pallor, coldness, wasting, and weakness should be studied by retrograde arteriography.[72]

102

ANTERIOR SCALENE SYNDROME

The chief symptoms of the anterior scalene syndrome are *numbness* and *tingling* of the arm, hands, and fingers. These sensations of the hand's "going to sleep" and of "pins and needles" are most prevalent during the early morning hours and frequently awaken the patient. Weakness in the fingers may be claimed, and when pain is present, it is described as deep, dull, and "aching."

Physical findings are minimal or absent. The findings are essentially subjective, and the examination consists of reproducing the symptoms by specific motions and positions. The scalene anticus test, also described as the "Adson test" (Fig. 78), consists of turning the head *to* the side of the symptoms, *extending* the head backward, abducting the arm, and taking a deep breath. By obliterating the radial pulse *in that arm* and *reduplicating the symptoms complained of* by the patient, the test is considered "positive."

The mechanism by which these maneuvers are considered to reproduce the symptoms is as follows: the rotated and extended position of the neck places the scalene muscle under tension, thus narrowing the angle between it and the first rib to which it attaches. Deep inspiration utilizes the scalenes as accessory inspiratory muscle and elevates the rib. The effects of these actions place traction and compression upon the neurovascular bundle.

Spasm of the scalene muscle implicated here may be caused from unusual exertion, posture, occupational stress, or prolonged emotional tension. More probably, scalene muscle spasm is secondary to cervical radiculitis due to spondylosis, diskogenic disease, or nerve root sleeve fibrosis.[73]

CLAVICULOCOSTAL SYNDROME

The neurovascular bundle may be compressed between the first rib and the clavicle at a point where the brachial plexus joins the subclavian artery and courses over the first rib (Fig. 79). The symptoms are similar to those of the anterior scalene syndrome, and the findings are minimal. Symptoms in this syndrome are reproduced by obliterating the radial pulse and by bringing the shoulders back and down. This postural maneuver is done, first, actively by the patient, then passively with downward pressure by the examiner.[74] A bruit, which can be heard when the vessels are compressed and disappears when they are released, is a good diagnostic confirmation.

The etiologic factors are posture, fatigue, trauma, and stress; thus the treatment is postural improvement and increase of muscle tone and endurance.

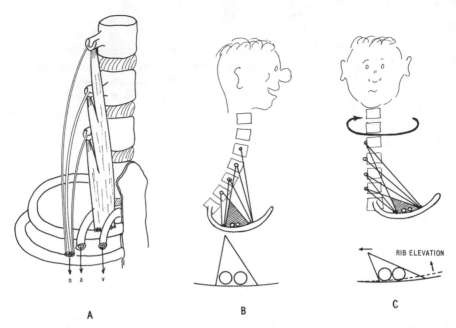

A   B   C

FIGURE 78. Scalene anticus syndrome. A. Relationship of the neurovascular bundle. The subclavian artery (a) passes behind the anterior scalene muscle, loops over the first rib, and is joined by the brachial plexus (n). The artery is separated from the subclavian vein (v) by the anterior scalene muscle. The median scalene muscle (not shown) lies behind the nerve (n). B. The triangle formed by the scalenes and the first rib. C. Distortion from turning the head toward the symptomatic side. Compression of the neurovascular bundle—the brachial plexus, the subclavian artery, and occasionally the subclavian vein—can be pictured from the test maneuver of the anticus scalene syndrome.

PECTORALIS MINOR SYNDROME

This syndrome is termed also the hyperabduction syndrome. The pectoralis minor muscle originates from the third, fourth, and fifth ribs anteriorly and inserts into the coracoid process of the scapula. The cords of the brachial plexus together with the axillary artery and vein descend over the first rib under cover of the pectoralis muscle (see Fig. 79).

The symptoms of numbness and tingling of the hand are caused by compression of the neurovascular bundle between the pectoralis minor muscle and the first rib and may be reduplicated by bringing the patient's arms overhead, abducted, and slightly backward. This position stretches the pectoralis minor muscle and narrows the space through which the neurovascular bundle traverses. The etiologic factors are similar to the scalene anticus and the claviculocostal syndromes; therefore, the treatment is similar.

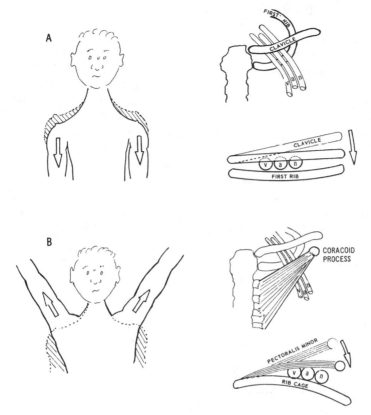

FIGURE 79. Claviculocostal and pectoralis minor syndromes. *A.* Claviculocostal syndrome. The neurovascular bundle is compressed between the clavicle and the first rib by retraction and depression of the shoulder girdles. *B.* Pectoralis minor syndrome. The neurovascular bundle may be compressed between the pectoralis minor and the rib cage by elevating the arms in a position of abduction and moving the arms behind the head.

SUPERIOR PULMONARY SULCUS TUMORS

Carcinoma of the lung or the Pancoast apical pulmonary tumor may first manifest itself by involvement of the brachial plexus. The pain is generally severe and diffusely located in the shoulder and arm. In addition to nerve root involvement, it is common for the tumor to involve the thoracic ganglion sympathetic chain and give rise to Horner's syndrome. There are usually associated general systemic signs and symptoms, positive chest x-ray films, and positive node biopsies. The specific treatment of the primary condition and for control of pain is surgery or irradiation. Follow-up treatment by physical medicine and rehabilitation consists of exercises and the use of indicated modalities.

SUPRASCAPULAR NERVE ENTRAPMENT

Pain in the shoulder can occur as a result of entrapment of the suprascapular nerve in its passage through the suprascapular foramen.[75] The course of the nerve is shown in Figure 49. It originates from C_5 and C_6, passes behind the brachial plexus to the upper border of the scapula, and passes through the suprascapular notch, where it is bridged over by the transverse scapular ligament. It then enters the supraspinatus fossa to supply the branches to the shoulder joint capsule, the acromioclavicular joint, and the supraspinatus and infraspinatus muscles. It is essentially a motor nerve; pain felt in its distribution is attributed to retrograde "myotome" sensory distribution, and is vague, deep, and poorly described. The posterior lateral aspect of the shoulder is described as the general area of painful sensation. Atrophy and weakness of the spinati muscles are frequent observations.

The nerve becomes fully stretched when the arm is held across the chest in *adduction*. Further adduction places stress upon the scapulothoracic joint and causes traction upon the nerve. Trauma is the usual mechanism, especially when there is an acromioclavicular separation allowing further scapular motion forward and medially.[76]

Diagnosis is made by eliciting the movement that initiated the pain, reproduction of the pain by forceful scapular movement forward and across the chest wall, failure to implicate another etiology or mechanism (negative evidence), and relief by a suprascapular nerve block.

Treatment is to treat any other associated problem, such as acromioclavicular separation, immobilization of scapula in position of no nerve tension, and repeated nerve blocks.

DORSAL SCAPULAR NERVE ENTRAPMENT

The dorsal scapular nerve innervates the rhomboids. It originates from the C_5 root and shortly after its origin perforates the medius scalene muscle. It is irritated by any condition that causes mechanical strain upon, or spasm of, the scalene musculature. The pain felt is dull, deep, and vague, along the medial edge of the scapula, because the nerve is principally a motor nerve. When the associated scalene conditions are favorably treated and all but the pain of the dorsal scapular nerve is relieved, surgical neurolysis is indicated.[76]

ARTERIOSCLEROTIC OCCLUSION

Arteriosclerotic occlusion produces a decreased blood flow and a reduced radial pulse. This conditions causes *claudication pain* when the patient exercises excessively, and it is relieved by rest. Systolic bruits are frequently heard. Innominate or subclavian aneurysm, with or without cervical rib compression, may mimic arteriosclerotic claudication. Arteriogram or venogram will confirm the clinical diagnosis.

CHAPTER 6

Sympathetic Referred Pain

Causalgia, reflex sympathetic dystrophy, and the shoulder-hand-finger syndrome have been grouped into a characteristic medical condition that may cause severe, intractable pain and progressive functional impairment and disability. The pain and ultimate disability is based on dysfunction of the sympathetic nervous system and thus the vascular system of the extremities.

The circulation of the upper extremity can be roughly divided into arterial and venous components.

1. The arterial circulation refers to cardiac pumping action, vascular tone, and gravitational forces, proceeding from the proximal to the distal portion of the extremity.
2. The venous return and lymphatic system carry back the circulation proximally by means of "pumps." The muscles of the hand and arm force the fluid in a centripetal direction through numerous valves in the venous system and through the lymphatic channels. Repeated elevation of the arm above the cardiac level allows gravity to aid this venous blood and lymphatic return.

The major pumps are located in the axilla and the hand (Fig. 80). These pumps require repeated movement of the shoulder girdle through adequate range of motion and repeated clenching and releasing of the fingers and wrist. Elevation of the arm above the shoulder level facilitates this centripetal flow.

The largest portion of the arterial supply is in the volar aspect of the hand, whereas most of the venous and lymphatic drainage is in the dorsal tissues of the hand.

Failure of these pumps to function adequately may lead to a painful and disabling condition termed *shoulder-hand-finger syndrome*. This

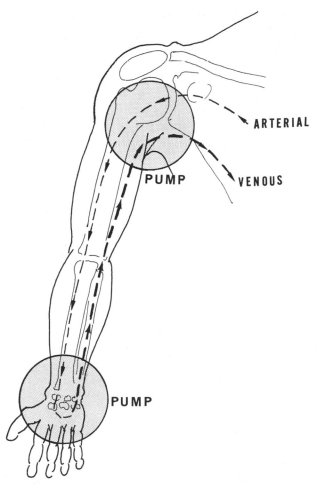

FIGURE 80. Venous lymphatic pumps of the upper extremity.

syndrome may be initiated at either of the pumping centers (the shoulder or the hand).

Reflex sympathetic dystrophies have been arbitrarily divided into major and minor classifications in which causalgia, phantom limb pain, and the central pains of the thalamus or thalamocortical tracts constitute the *major* dystrophies. All other causalgias related to trauma or disease are considered *minor dystrophies.* The shoulder-hand-finger syndrome is in this latter category.

Causalgia is essentially a symptom complex that has gradually become a distinct disease entity. The causalgic aspect of the complex is appreciation of a persistent "burning pain," usually following trauma.

Pain, if it appears, usually arises shortly after injury but may actually occur after the initial injury has healed or subsided. This causalgic pain is vague, diffuse, and poorly delineated. It corresponds to no peripheral radicular or dermatome pattern.

"Burning" pain is associated with vasospastic or vasodilatory phenomena and is usually described by the patient as severe to excruciating. The initial incident or injury may be minor, but once initiated it may progress to impairment with irreversible tissue changes.

A voluminous literature has evolved regarding causalgia, with the introduction of terms such as reflex sympathetic dystrophy, Sudeck's atrophy, traumatic vasospasm, postinfarction sclerodactylia, posttraumatic osteoporosis, chronic traumatic edema, and shoulder-hand-finger syndrome. In this syndrome there is a resultant immobilizing of the involved part, resulting in chronic edema, fibrosis, joint contracture, and muscle and bone atrophy[77] (Fig. 81).

The inciting traumata that provoke the reflex sympathetic dystrophy are varied and frequently nonapparent. They include cardiovascular disease such as hemiplegia or coronary ischemia, cervical disk disease, mechanical trauma, prolonged bed rest, or even an incident as innocuous as an intramuscular injection. The inciting factor may be a subacute peritendinitis of the shoulder, a calcific tendinitis, subluxation, "frozen shoulder," or a bicipital tendinitis. No overt cause may have been discovered. *A pain must have existed. Immobilization of the part must have followed. Sympathetic vasomotor reaction must have been invoked.*

PATHOPHYSIOLOGIC MECHANISMS

The pathologic changes discernible in the extremity are frequently insufficient to account for the severity of the symptoms. The peripheral and central pathways of pain in this causalgic state are not well understood neurophysiologically. The sympathetic nervous system is universally implicated, and many pathways are described; but all theories are based on the unproven presence of *afferent* pain fibers in the sympathetic nervous system.

The accepted pathways of sensation are shown in Figure 82A. The segmental nerve arises from various tissues: cutaneous, subcutaneous, tendons, joints, periosteum, and skeletal muscle. Impulses proceed proximally through the anterior and posterior primary divisions of the segmental nerve through the posterior root ganglion and enter the cord to take various pathways depending on the type of sensation transmitted. The pain and thermal fibers, immediately upon entering the cord, synapse at the same segmental level and ascend in the posterior lateral tract to a level several segments higher. Some of the pain

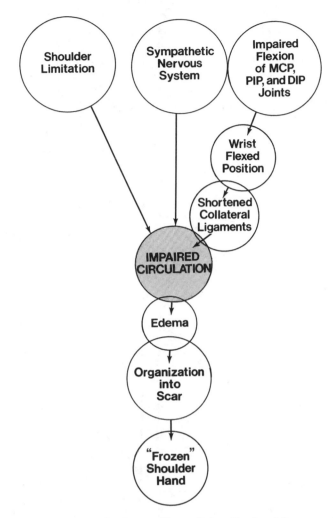

FIGURE 81. Sequences leading to "frozen" shoulder-hand-finger syndrome.

and temperature fibers decussate and ascend the cord in the lateral spinothalamic tract. The ipsilateral posterior column transmits position sensation, and the anterior spinothalamic columns, tactile sensation.

Pain sensation entering the cord from the sensory ganglion excites the internuncial pool in the gray matter of the cord. A reverberating cycle is initiated that excites the anterior horn cells and causes a motor response in the peripheral musculature. A simultaneous excitation of the lateral horn cells occurs, which causes a sympathetic vasomotor and sudomotor response. This cycle at the segmental level involves

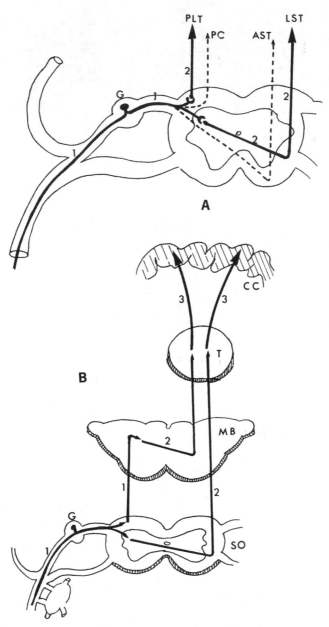

FIGURE 82. Neuron pathways of pain. A. The course of sensory fibers in a segmental nerve with its ganglion in the dorsal root (G). Upon entrance into the cord, the fibers ascend on the same side in the posterior lateral tract (PLT) and decussate to cross into the lateral spinothalamic tract; 2 indicates secondary neurons. The posterior column (PC) transmits position sense; AST conveys tactile sensation. B. 1 = first-stage neurons to the cord; 2 = second-stage neurons through the midbrain (MB) into the thalamus (T); 3 = third-stage neurons, the thalamocortical pathways to the cerebral cortex (CC).

first-order neurons. The internuncial pool and the pathways from it to the thalamus constitute the *neurons* of the *second order.* The *third-order neuron* connects the thalamus to the cerebral cortex through the corticothalamic cycle.

This three-neuron cycle *does not* fully explain the observable clinical aspect of vasodilatation in the causalgic state. The "cycle" theory which would cause excitation of the lateral cells with sympathetic release would cause vasoconstriction, not dilatation, and dilatation occurs peripherally.[78] This theory also does not explain fully the relief of pain from sympathectomy, unless the presence of *afferent* fibers (antidromic) in the sympathetic ganglia and trunks is accepted. Figure 83A shows the accepted flow of sympathetic nerve impulses. Figure 83B depicts the antidromic flow of sympathetic impulses coupled with the cycle of internuncial pool stimuli, which now has acceptable recognition.

Confirmation of afferent fibers in the sympathetic nerve ganglia and trunks has been advanced. Retrograde degeneration following section of the *rami communicantes* indicates the presence of afferent fibers.[79] In laboratory experiments extensive bilateral dorsal rhizotomies (eliminating sensory nerve roots) and unilateral sympathectomies allowed the animals to perceive pain on the side where the sympathetic fibers remained. It was concluded that *afferent fibers exist capable of transmitting pain sensations through the sympathetic trunks along the segmental nerves to the spinal cord.*[80]

Treatment of the causalgic state depends upon the duration of the painful stimulus, the duration of the reverberating internuncial cycle, and the order (first, second, or third) of neurons involved.

DIAGNOSIS

The shoulder is involved first as a rule, but the painful hand may precede a specific aspect of the causalgic state. In 1897, Osler described shoulder disability in patients suffering from angina pectoris, and in 1948 the complex of shoulder and hand abnormalities on a neurovascular basis was formulated.[81] Regardless of the site or source of the pain sensation, the syndrome follows a specific pattern.

The syndrome occurs with equal frequency in either or both shoulders and, except when caused by coronary occlusion, is most frequent in women. The shoulder is generally involved first, but the painful hand may precede the shoulder. Three stages of the complex are recognized.

The shoulder becomes "stiff," limited in its range of motion, and may proceed to a "frozen shoulder." Even in cases following a myocardial infarction, the shoulder initially resembles the pericapsulitis

113

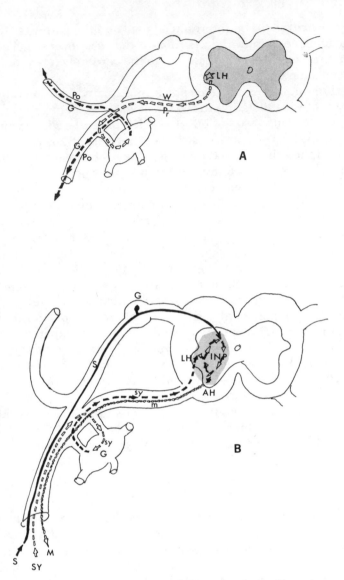

FIGURE 83. *A.* The accepted direction of the sympathetic fibers in a segmental peripheral nerve. The preganglionic myelinated white (W) nerve (Pr), the postganglionic (Po) unmyelinated nerve that leave as gray (G) fibers through the gray ramus of the ganglion, and proceed distally within the common peripheral nerve. *B.* The afferent pathways along the sympathetic nerve. The cycle of the sensory nerve root (S) excites the intranuncial pool (INP), which in turn excites afferent sympathetic nerves (SY) and afferent motor impulses (M). LH indicates lateral horn cells; AH, anterior horn.

from other causes. Tenderness about the shoulder is diffuse and not localized to a specific tendon or bursal area. The duration of the initial

114

shoulder stage, before the hand component begins, is extremely variable. The shoulder may be "stiff" for several months before the hand becomes involved, or both may occur simultaneously.

The hand and fingers become diffusely swollen. At first the edema is pitting and may be relieved by prolonged elevation of the arm. This edema is predominantly noted on the dorsum of the hand and usually is noted over the metacarpophalangeal and proximal interphalangeal joints (Fig. 84). The skin over the knuckles becomes puffy and loses the normal creases. The hand becomes boggy and painful. As the edema forms under the extensor tendons flexion becomes increasingly more limited. The collateral ligaments, which must elongate to permit flexion of the metacarpophalangeal joints, become shortened and thus prevent or limit full flexion (Fig. 85).

Less pumping action is permitted, and with the limited shoulder action allowing no ability to elevate the arm above shoulder level, both pumps are restricted.

The skin gradually becomes shiny and atrophic. The edema-containing protein converts into a diffuse, cobweb-like tissue that adheres to the tendons and joint capsules and prevents further movement.

The joints undergo disuse atrophy of the cartilage, and the capsule thickens. The bones undergo diffuse osteoporosis. The ultimate hand posture resembles the *intrinsic minus hand* (Fig. 86) due to stiffening of the metacarpophalangeal joint in extension with the tenodesis flexor action flexing the phalanges.

The evolution of the shoulder-hand-finger syndrome can be itemized in the following sequence (see Fig. 81):

1. Impairment of the hand-arm-shoulder venous and lymphatic circulation.
2. Shoulder limitation from numerous causes leading to ultimate contracture ("frozen shoulder").
3. Metacarpophalangeal limitation due to edema and restricting, contracted collateral ligaments.
4. Wrist in a restricted, flexed position.
5. Sympathetic nervous system involvement.

Sympathetic nervous system involvement may be totally absent, initially absent, or may be primary in the causation of the shoulder-hand-finger syndrome. Some deny the necessity of this component,[82] based on the fact that the syndrome is rarely seen in people who are less than 40 years old, which is when sympathetic nervous system abnormalities are most prevalent. Causes considered necessary for sympathetic nervous system involvement are frequently not present. When present, the resultant clinical entity is termed *reflex sympa-*

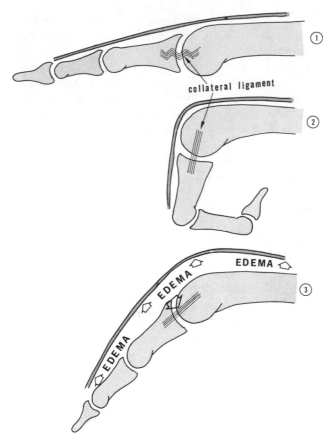

FIGURE 84. Finger changes in the hand-shoulder syndrome. 1. Normal extension of the metacarpophalangeal joint with relaxed collateral ligament. 2. Normal flexion of the metacarpophalangeal joint with the collaterals becoming taut. 3. Edema on the dorsum of the hand elevates the extensor tendons and prevents flexion. The collateral ligaments are never fully elongated and develop contracture. This further limits the "pump action" of the flexion of the hand.

thetic dystrophy syndrome or *causalgia.*

Reflex sympathetic dystrophy syndrome has the following classic signs and symptoms:

1. Pain and swelling in an extremity
2. Trophic skin changes of that extremity which include:
   a. Skin atrophy
   b. Skin pigmentary changes
   c. Hyperhidrosis
   d. Hypertrichosis

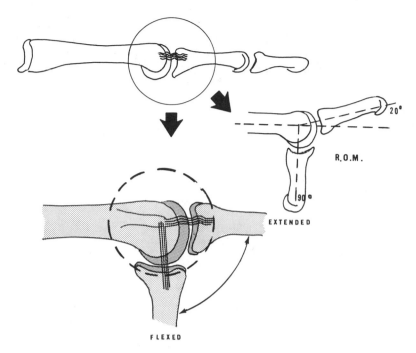

FIGURE 85. Normal flexion-extension of the metacarpophalangeal joints. Due to the elliptical shape of the head of the metacarpals, the collateral ligaments are slack with finger extension and taut when the fingers are flexed.

    e. Nail changes
3. Signs and symptoms of vasomotor instability
4. Pain and limited range of motion of the ipsilateral shoulder
5. Precipitating events such as stroke, trauma, and myocardial infarction

Most reflex sympathetic dystrophy syndromes are unilateral, but 20 to 35 percent are bilateral. Studies of reflex dystrophy by oscillography, plethysmography, skin temperature, and venous gas determinations reveal increased blood flow and increased venous oxygen. In reflex sympathetic dystrophy syndrome, there are *no* characteristic pathologic tissue changes. Ultimately there is radiologic evidence of periarticular soft tissue swelling and patchy osteoporosis, but these changes are similar to changes noted in prolonged immobilization.[83]

The shoulder-hand-finger syndrome, which is a variant of the reflex sympathetic dystrophy syndrome, has been considered to evolve into three stages. These stages need not be in the same sequence, but the third is usually the residual stage. The stages are not necessarily as specific or as clearly delineated as stated:

117

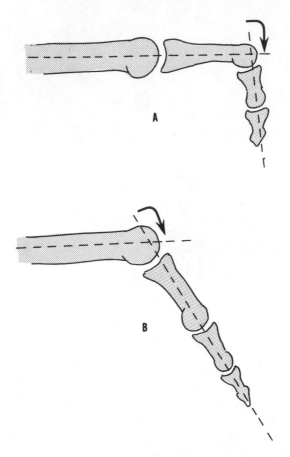

FIGURE 86. Hand patterns. *A* depicts the hand that resembles the "intrinsic minus hand." The proximal phalanx remains extended with tenodesis action flexing the distal phalanges. *B* resembles the "intrinsic minus hand," with all phalanges extended but with the metacarpophalangeal joint flexed.

1. Limited shoulder range of motion with or without pain. The hand has swelling limited initially to the dorsum of the fingers, knuckles, and wrist. Edema is not usually of the pitting variety but is firm. The skin loses its normal wrinkles and becomes shiny. Full flexion of the fingers and all their joints becomes limited. The wrist tends to assume a flexed posture. The skin of the hand may be pale and cool or assume a pink hue. The skin is usually moist with small bubbles of perspiration. In certain cases, the skin is excessively hypersensitive to touch, pressure, movement, or temperature variations. The elbow usually shows no limitation or pain. The wrist is usually exquisitely painful when extended and also has dorsal edema and tenderness.

2. Shoulder pain subsides and shoulder range may increase. Residual restriction of movement in both the active and passive ranges may persist, but this limitation is usually less painful. Edema of the hand subsides, but the fingers become stiffer. The skin assumes a pale, atrophic appearance. Hair appears coarser, as do the nails. Sensitivity decreases. Osteoporosis can now be visualized on x-ray.
3. There is progressive atrophy of the bones, skin, and muscles. Limitation of hands, wrists, and fingers increases, leaving the hand painless but in a useless, atrophied, clawed position.

ETIOLOGY

Initial causalgic pain is mediated through the large delta fibers which transmit brief, sharp, pricking, localized pain which, when elicited, promptly causes withdrawal. The secondary pain is delayed and mediated through the small-diameter fibers that are slow-conducting. This is the pain that is persistent and of a burning quality. In causalgia, the macroscopic and microscopic appearance of the involved nerve lesions is not different from lesions which do not cause burning pain.

Electrical stimulation of the distal end of the divided nerves in a peripheral nerve injury with causalgia releases neurokinin, a substance that is a vasodilator. Neurokinin, which can be retrieved from the tissues, will cause a burning pain when injected into normal tissues. In causalgia, it is probable that neurokinin is liberated, but this has not been verified.

TREATMENT

Early vigorous treatment of the shoulder-hand syndrome offers the only promise of recovery.

The stiff shoulder should be treated, utilizing all medications and modalities to improve range of motion. Disuse must be avoided, since it is the predominant instigator of the shoulder phases. Where and when possible, the underlying cause must be treated as in diaphragmatic irritation, myocardial infarction, and gallbladder disease. Regardless of the underlying source of pain, the shoulder and hand must receive early active treatment.

During the phase of pain relief from the stellate block, gentle, cautious, but positive active physical therapy must be started. Massage, hot packs, whirlpool, and even ice packs are usually poorly tolerated. Cool packs about 70° F are usually most soothing. Local irritation may stimulate more sympathetic fibers.

119

Active exercises of the shoulder and hand must be instituted as soon and as energetically as the medical condition permits. Stasis must be prevented and active circulation stimulated, even though sympathetic vasospasm exists. Movement of the hand and shoulder "pumps" the venous blood from the fingers toward the axilla, which, coupled with an elevated overhead arm position, decreases distal edema. The major "pumping" action occurs at the metacarpophalangeal joints and the axilla; therefore edema of the dorsum of the hand impairs the meta-carpophalangeal pumping action.

The hand and fingers must be kept adequate for their pumping role. The wrist must be kept flexible so that flexion-extension motion of the fingers is maintained. In a wrist that is permitted to remain flexed, the finger flexor tendons are restricted; therefore flexion at the meta-carpophalangeal and phalangeal joints is impaired. The "pumping action" of the hand, which occurs predominantly at the metacarpo-phalangeal joints, is lost. The metacarpal and collateral ligaments are placed under tension when the hand is flexed, and these must be kept fully extendible.

In the early dystrophic phase of the hand, sympathetic procaine block must be instituted immediately. Done early, these blocks are both diagnostic and therapeutic. An effective block may wear off in 24 hours and have to be repeated. One block may clear the condition completely, or a second block may need to be performed 5 to 7 days later. The controversy as to whether repeated blocks should be done upon cessation of pain is an individual decision. Regardless of cessa-tion of pain, repeated blocks should be considered when there is continuation of vasomotor and sudomotor changes (Fig. 87).

An effective stellate block is so judged if there is (1) pain relief; (2) Horner's syndrome (miosis, enophthalmos, and ptosis; anhidriosis, injected conjunctiva, slightly flushed face, and blocked nostrils are also consistent); or (3) a marked rise in the skin temperature. The technique of performing a stellate block is well documented in the literature.[84]

More permanent benefit from sympathetic intervention can be prognosticated as:

1. Good
   a. if one block gives total relief;
   b. if one block reduces pain to a tolerable level;
   c. if the first block is effective with each subsequent block being "better."
2. Poor
   a. if the first block is effective but each subsequent block is less effective;

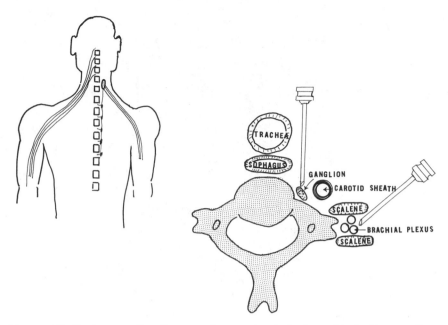

FIGURE 87. Technique of stellate ganglion or brachial plexus block. For a stellate ganglion nerve block, the trachea is moved to one side and the needle enters between it and the carotid artery to the vertebral body. The needle then is moved slightly lateral to the body, and 3 to 5 cc of the anesthetic agent is administered. Aspiration must always precede infiltration of the anesthetic agent.

    b. if the block is only effective during the duration of the anesthetic agent but there is no residual benefit after the agent wears off.

If the decision is made, by the physician or at the request of the patient, not to administer a stellate chemical block, oral or intramuscular steroids can be effectively substituted. A usual dose of triamcinolone, 100 mg daily, or cortisone, 200 mg daily, for 14 to 16 days may be of great benefit. The precautions of administering steroids must obviously be observed.

In addition to oral, intramuscular medication or stellate chemical blocks, other physical therapeutic modalities must be instituted, including all the exercise methods of treatment advocated for the painful and limited shoulder. For the hand and fingers, vasoconstrictive techniques to reduce the edema must be instituted. Elastic bandaging, wrapping the fingers with twine (Fig. 88), or use of a Jobst vasopneumatic compressive device can be of value.

Elevation of the arm above shoulder level, achievable range of motion permitting, is generally attempted. This may be accomplished by

121

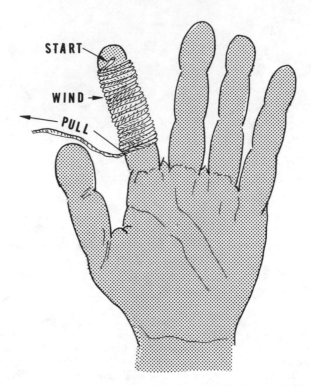

FIGURE 88. Removal of finger edema. Each finger is firmly wrapped with a heavy twine, beginning at the tip and moving toward the webbing. This procedure should be performed several times daily and can frequently be done by the patient, using his uninvolved upper extremity.

placing the arm and hand on a pillow or by suspending it from overhead equipment (Fig. 89).

PSYCHIATRIC ASPECTS

The full psychiatric implications of reflex sympathetic dystrophy are beyond the scope of this text, but the subject cannot be dismissed altogether from this discussion.

The designation of *periarthritic personality* is used repeatedly throughout the literature[31] and varies in meaning from a primary inciting cause to the personality resulting from persistent, unrelenting pain.[1,84] The question has been raised whether the causalgic state is a purely psychogenic phenomenon complicated by compensation-induced voluntary immobilization and aggravated by conversion hysteria or pathologic malingering.[85]

The sensation of pain and the patient's reaction to pain are associ-

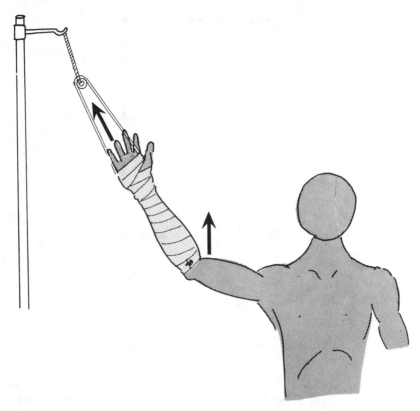

FIGURE 89. Antigravity treatment of the edematous extremity. The hand and arm are wrapped, distal to proximal, with an elastic bandage. The hand held by the webrill is then suspended overhead. This position drains the edema and maintains shoulder range of motion with the elbow extended.

ated with a state of anguish, displeasure, and fear. In the early phase of the shoulder or the hand component of minor reflex dystrophy, movement is avoided because of pain. Interest, judicious sympathy, and encouragement are necessary to initiate and maintain the active movement so important in the recovery process. Early interruption of the "cycle" by stellate blocks prevents the internuncial reverberation and progression to the second and third neuronal levels where treatment by any means becomes increasingly ineffectual and, in fact, ultimately useless.

Continuous sensory *input* reaching the hypothalamus increases its reactivity, and stimuli of lesser and lesser intensity respond with exaggerated sympathetic outbursts.[86] It behooves the treating physician to interrupt the pain cycle early and forcefully. Arresting the pathophysiologic manifestations early and preventing progression of

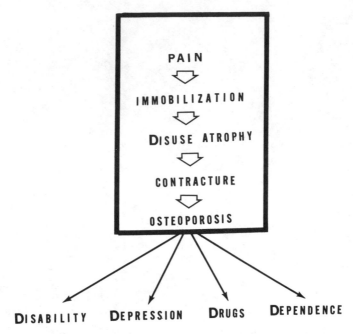

FIGURE 90. The "five Ds" resulting from pain.

symptoms minimize the psychologic factors.[18,87] Whether the psychologic factors are primary or secondary is of incidental importance when the concern is to prevent permanent functional disability (Fig. 90).

Pain perception is subjective and results from the way the sensory impulses reaching the cortical level are processed and interpreted. Pain can be influenced by drugs with an analgesic or a hypnotic action, but it has been shown to be influenced also by the patient's attitude and suggestibility.[44]

The treatment of pain and its effect, therefore, are multifaceted: (1) interrupt, eliminate, or minimize the sensory-pain impulse by all means; (2) prevent secondary manifestations that may become initiators of pain as well as complicate the primary factors; (3) elevate the pain tolerance by suggestion, sympathy, and encouragement; (4) alter the interpretation of pain by drugs or psychotherapy; and (5) remove the patient's motivation to be disabled, whether it is a monetary compensation or a psychogenic, hysterical manifestation.

CHAPTER 7

Traumatic Pain

Shoulder dislocations at the glenohumeral joint occur anteriorly in 90 percent of shoulder dislocations. The remaining 10 percent dislocate posteriorly. The prevalence of anterior dislocations is attributed to the anatomic weakness of the anterior aspect of the joint.

Brief review of the anatomy of the glenohumeral joint, described in Chapter 1, reveals the capsule to be thin and loose. The capsule is reinforced anteriorly by folds called the glenohumeral ligaments. These ligaments attach from the humerus and fan out to attach to the superior anterior aspect of the glenoid fossa, partly to the glenoid labrum, and partly to a portion of the bone of the scapula. An opening in the capsule frequently exists between the superior and middle glenohumeral ligaments, termed the foramen of Weitbrecht. This may be a frank perforation or may be covered by a thin layer of capsule. The articular cavity connects with the subscapular fossa through this opening. The humeral head dislocates through this opening, and dislocations may recur due to fraying or actual destruction of the middle glenohumeral ligament (Fig. 91).

In dislocations the glenoid labrum may be partially or completely detached with the tear occurring in the anteroinferior aspect.[88] If the concept is accepted that the glenoid labrum contains *no* fibrocartilage but is merely a redundant fibrous fold of the anterior capsule that disappears when the humerus is externally rotated, this "pouch" invites dislocation. The humeral head can protrude into this pouch, especially if an anatomic variant of the middle humeral ligament exists.

There are four types of dislocation, the most common being the subcoracoid. The subclavicular and subglenoid types are less frequent and may be a progression of the subcoracoid type. All anterior types can change into any other of the anterior types. The type of dislocation is so termed depending upon the site of the humeral head in relation

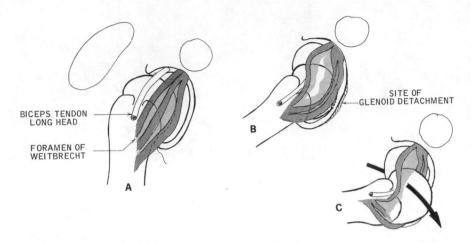

BICEPS TENDON
LONG HEAD

FORAMEN OF
WEITBRECHT

A

B

SITE OF
GLENOID DETACHMENT

C

FIGURE 91. Anterior capsule, glenohumeral ligaments, and avenue of anterior shoulder dislocation. *A.* The three folds of the anterior capsule forming the glenohumeral ligaments that attach from the anterior ridge of the humerus to the glenoid fossa. *B.* A tear is shown in the area between the superior and middle ligament (foramen of Weitbrecht), which may be covered by a thin capsule or may be a direct opening. *C.* As the head of the humerus moves forward and downward, it emerges through the opening.

to the glenoid seat when the diagnosis is made. The fourth type—the posterior or subspinous—is rare (Fig. 92).

Primary anterior dislocations occur with equal frequency regardless of age, but *recurrence* of dislocation is highest in the young (teens and twenties) and decreases after age 45. There is less recurrence in those cases in which the primary dislocation was severe as a result of the greater hemorrhage and therefore the greater scar formation in healing.

MECHANISM OF DISLOCATION

Anterior dislocations result from abduction–external rotation injuries. Trauma usually "catches" the muscles that protect the joint unprepared, or is of sufficient force to overwhelm the muscles. In younger people the anterior glenohumeral ligaments "give," whereas in older people the posterior supports, the greater tuberosity, or the supraspinatus and infraspinatus tendons tear, permitting the head of the humerus to "roll" over the anterior rim. The capsule and glenohumeral ligaments remain intact (Fig. 93).

A frequent explanation offered for anterior dislocation is depicted in Figure 94. As stated by Codman,[1] "the capacity for rotation will be less as the arm ascends until, in complete elevation, tuberosities and processes will be locked in a fixed position." To elevate the arm fully in

126

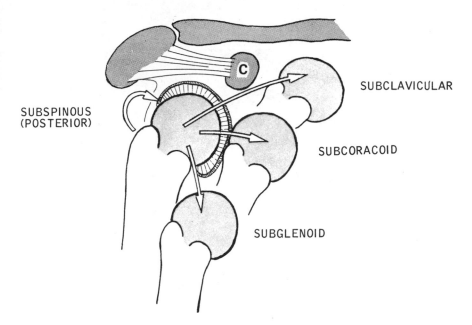

SUBSPINOUS
(POSTERIOR)

SUBCLAVICULAR

SUBCORACOID

SUBGLENOID

FIGURE 92. Four types of shoulder dislocation. The subcoracoid dislocation is the most frequent and the subspinous (posterior), the least common. All three anterior dislocations—the subcoracoid, the subglenoid, and the subclavicular—may alternate. The type designated depends upon the position of the humeral head in relation to the glenoid seat at the time of diagnosis.

the coronal plane, the arm must be externally rotated. In the sagittal plane internal rotation of the arm is necessary to achieve full elevation. If either rotational adjustments are violated and force is applied to accomplish elevation, a fulcrum is created whereby the distal force causes downward and anterior displacement of the proximal head.

The mechanism of primary dislocations and recurrent dislocations was considered to differ in past literature, but present concepts imply a similar mechanism with recurrence being easier as a result of the primary dislocation having been *incorrectly treated*.[89]

The method of dislocation is most often caused by a fall on the outstretched arm (Fig. 94, parts 1–4). The trauma drives the head forward against the anterior capsule.[9]

A less frequent cause of *redislocation* is the occurrence of bony lesions at the time of primary dislocation in which there is fragmentation of the anterior bony ridge or a posterior lateral defect, the so-called compression notch of Hermodsson.[90,91] Special x-ray techniques are required to see this defect.[92] The mechanism is alleged to be a pivoting motion around a strong coracohumeral ligament that causes compression of the posterolateral portion of the humeral head against

127

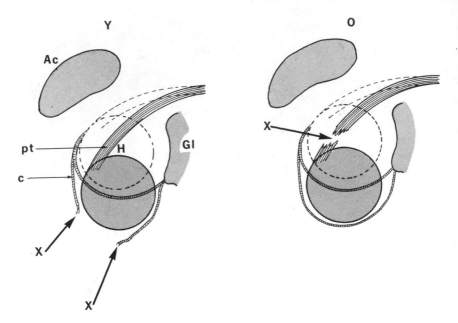

FIGURE 93. Relationship of age of patient to mechanism of anterior dislocation. Y shows the normal relationship, in the young, of the head of the humerus (H) to the glenoid fossa (Gl) with intact posterior tissues (pt) consisting of the supra- and infraspinatus tendons attached to the greater tuberosity. The capsule (c) is intact, albeit thin and loose. The mechanism of dislocation in the young causes tear through the anterior capsule (*X arrows*). O. In older people, the posterior tissues tear (*X arrow*), or the greater tuberosity avulses. In this latter mechanism the head of the humerus "rolls" over the anterior rim of the glenoid but does not tear the anterior capsule.

the sharp posterior rim of the glenoid, so that a compression defect results (Fig. 95).

Posterior dislocation, though rare, must be recognized early; otherwise, reduction becomes difficult, and postreduction complications may result. The posterior dislocation finds the head behind the scapula, usually caused by trauma to the *flexed, abducted* arm. The trauma is usually a blow to the front of the shoulder, causing forceful backward movement of the head. Posterior dislocation may occur during convulsion.

DIAGNOSIS OF DISLOCATION

In anterior dislocation, since the humeral head does not occupy its usual position, the round appearance of the shoulder is lost. The acromion appears to be unusually prominent because of the hollow space beneath, caused by the absence of the humerus. All movements are limited and painful. Because the head is "locked" in a medial

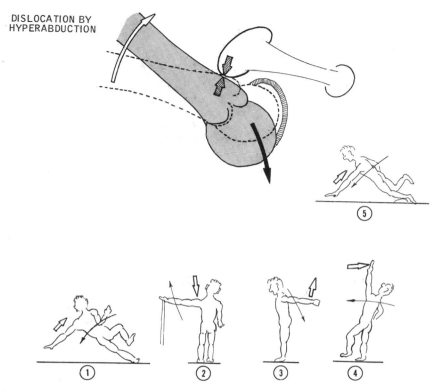

DISLOCATION BY
HYPERABDUCTION

FIGURE 94. Mechanism of dislocation: "hyperextension theory." Abduction with the humerus in internal rotation or forward flexion with the arm in external rotation becomes limited by the acromial arch. Forceful elevation when this point of impingement has been reached uses the arch as a fulcrum and dislocates the proximal head by causing it to descend and move forward.

position, the lower end of the humerus "sticks out," and the elbow will not reach the trunk. If the dislocation proceeds to a subglenoid position, the arm may be locked in full abducted position (*luxatio erecta*).

Posterior dislocations find the arm fixed in internal rotation, and any motion attempting external rotation is impossible. Regaining the neutral position may be prevented. The coracoid is prominent, and frequently the humerus can be palpated posteriorly under the scapular spine.

X-rays of anterior dislocation are diagnostic, but routine views in cases of posterior dislocation may reveal little or no abnormality. Routine anteroposterior views in posterior dislocation may be suggestive, but auxiliary and tangential views are necessary to confirm the diagnosis.

Persistent pain following a shoulder dislocation may mean an asso-

129

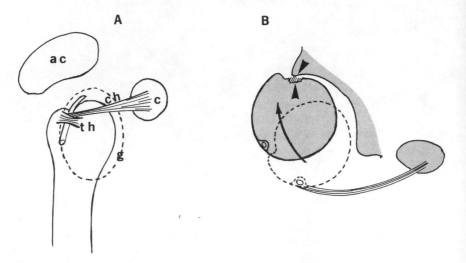

FIGURE 95. Intra-articular fracture in recurrent shoulder dislocation ("notch lesion of Hermodsson"). A strong coracohumeral ligament acts as a pivot point that causes the humerus to compress against the posterior rim of the glenoid and cause a compression fracture (indenture) in the posterolateral aspect of the humerus.

ciated cuff tear, a glenoid labrum tear, or an avulsion fracture of the greater tuberosity. Exploration may be needed for absolute diagnosis of cuff or glenoid labrum tears, whereas x-ray usually reveals the tuberosity fracture.

TREATMENT

Closed reductions of uncomplicated anterior dislocations are usually possible. Gentle traction and anesthesia may be necessary with the patient lying prone on a table and the arm dangling. Reduction usually can be accomplished. The original Hippocratic method is still practiced. Traction is applied to the arm along the side of the body while the surgeon's stocking foot is placed in the axilla as counter-pressure. While traction is applied, the arm is brought in toward the body; thus the head is levered outward around the fulcrum created by the manipulator's foot.

No discussion of closed reduction of an anterior dislocation would be complete without mentioning Kocher's method,[93] depicted in Figure 96 and discussed in the legend. A certain skill and definite gentleness are necessary in this maneuver. Frequently, reduction may be accomplished and not realized by the surgeon. A "click," usually considered reduction, may merely be a change from one form of dislocation to another, not a complete reduction. The external rotation phase

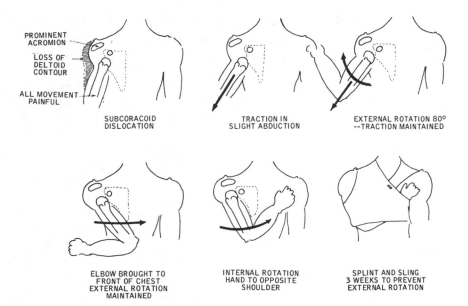

PROMINENT ACROMION
LOSS OF DELTOID CONTOUR
ALL MOVEMENT PAINFUL

SUBCORACOID DISLOCATION

TRACTION IN SLIGHT ABDUCTION

EXTERNAL ROTATION 80° --TRACTION MAINTAINED

ELBOW BROUGHT TO FRONT OF CHEST EXTERNAL ROTATION MAINTAINED

INTERNAL ROTATION HAND TO OPPOSITE SHOULDER

SPLINT AND SLING 3 WEEKS TO PREVENT EXTERNAL ROTATION

FIGURE 96. Kocher manipulation for closed treatment of dislocation. All movements should be done smoothly and gently. Traction should be maintained constantly. Once reduced, the arm is splinted for 3 weeks to prevent external rotation.

of the maneuver may tear the subscapularis or even cause a spiral fracture of the humerus.

After reduction, the arm is bound to the chest wall in a sling support to prevent external rotation. During this 3-week splinting, *the wrist and fingers should be actively and frequently exercised.* After 3 weeks the splint is removed, and *active* exercises to strengthen *adduction,* internal rotation, and abduction in the internally rotated position of the humerus should be started, supervised, and encouraged. *No active assisted exercises and no passive stretching exercises should be done.* Isometric active exercises are very valuable here.

If an avulsion of the supraspinatus tendon or an avulsion fracture of the greater tuberosity of the humerus exists, the arm must be splinted to hold the humerus in an *abducted, externally rotated, and forward flexed position* horizontally. This position is maintained in an airplane splint.

Reduction of a posterior dislocation is usually done under general anesthesia. Gentle traction, in the line of the humerus, with simultaneous pressure exerted from behind the head, will bring the head into the cradle of the glenoid. *External* rotation of the humerus may be necessary to reduce the dislocation. Once reduction of the arm is accomplished, the arm is splinted in a plaster cast in *external* rotation and a slight abduction, with the humerus (elbow) slightly behind the midline of the trunk. In 3 weeks, *active* exercises are begun, with avoidance of any passive stretching, and stress is placed on *external* abduction exercises. Full range is usually achieved in 6 weeks.

Dislocations of long duration in which there are glenoid changes, old unrecognized dislocations, cuff tears, or unreduced avulsion fractures may require open reduction. The surgical techniques are beyond the scope of this text.

In older people who suffer an anterior dislocation (see Fig. 93), the tear of the posterior structures prolongs the convalescence, and a degree of stiffness, pain and disability is the rule. The treatment of older patients, therefore, differs from that of younger people in that, with redislocation being rare but stiffness and pain being frequent, prolonged immobilization *must be avoided,* so usually within 10 days pendular exercises are begun. Surgical intervention for recurrent anterior dislocation attempts any procedure that will buttress the anterior capsule of the joint or will prevent external rotation. In posterior dislocation transplant of the subscapularis may be necessary.

Open reduction of avulsion fractures of the greater tuberosity is indicated when closed reduction has left a fragment displacement of 1 cm or more. Screw fixation of the fragment is necessary. A lesser displacement with intact periosteum will heal after approximation by closed reduction.

The complications of dislocation, other than tear, of the supraspinatus tendon and avulsion fracture of the greater tuberosity include nerve and blood vessel injury. Nerve injuries to the brachial plexus usually involve the posterior cord (radial, axillary, subscapular, and thoracodorsal nerves); thus, since the muscles innervated are the deltoid (*axillary nerve*), triceps (*radial nerve*), latissimus dorsi (*thoracodorsal nerve*), and the teres major (*subscapular nerve*), there is weakness of the extensors and elevators, and internal rotation of the arm (Fig. 97). Whereas nerve lesions are rare in fractures of the upper end of the humerus, they are frequent in dislocation. The axillary nerve can be damaged as it circles around the surgical neck of the humerus and thus cause paresis or paralysis of the deltoid muscle.[40]

The axillary blood vessels may be injured, with the hand becoming blue, then cold and pale—a pulse deficit—and swelling being noted in the axilla. Early recognition and emergency surgical intervention are mandatory.[94]

ACROMIOCLAVICULAR LESIONS

The acromioclavicular joint as the site of pain in the shoulder is frequently overlooked. This joint is subject to the various arthritides

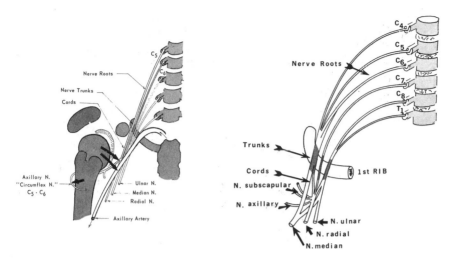

FIGURE 97. Schematic brachial plexus. Emphasis (*shaded area*) is placed on the posterior cord forming the radial, axillary, and subscapular nerves, this being the cord most often involved in shoulder separation.

(osteo-, rheumatoid, tuberculous, and traumatic), to osteochondritis, and to numerous traumata causing contusion, sprain, and separation.[95]

This joint is relatively weak and inflexible for the constant burden and repeated stresses it bears. Heavy laborers who lift objects overhead or carry weights on their shoulders and participants in competitive contact sports have frequent stress applied to the acromion or the acromioclavicular joint. Whether the stresses to this joint are direct or indirect, the mechanism of trauma is identical.

The mechanism of acromioclavicular joint disruption has been well documented.[96,97] Force applied to the acromion or the glenohumeral joint from above causes the scapula to rotate around the coracoid, which becomes a fulcrum. The superior and inferior acromioclavicular ligaments, being intrinsically weak, give way and the joint dislocates (Fig. 98). A downward force of greater intensity lowers the clavicle upon the first rib, and the rib becomes the fulcrum. The coracoclavicular and the coracoacromial ligaments tear (see Figs. 2 and 30), causing a complete acromioclavicular separation. Sufficient force can fracture the clavicle.

Incomplete subluxations may tear the intra-articular meniscus (see Fig. 29) and lead to degenerative, painful arthritis of the acromioclavicular joint. Muscular action upon the joint enhances the dislocating forces that cause acromioclavicular dislocation. The upper trapezius muscle fibers elevate the clavicle, while the deltoid muscle, supplementing the gravity effect of the weight of the arm, pulls down upon the acromion (see Fig. 33).

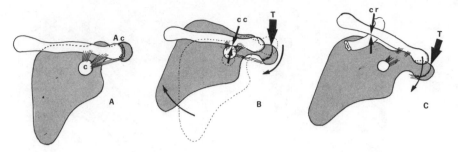

FIGURE 98. Mechanism of acromioclavicular separation. *A*. The normal relationship of the clavicle to the scapula with intact coracoclavicular and coracoacromial ligaments. *B*. The rotation of the scapula with the coracoid (c) acting as a fulcrum under the clavicle. Trauma (T) is from above. Contact of coracoid to clavicle is at arrows cc. *C*. Further force from T causes the clavicle to descend further and impinge upon the first rib at point cr, causing the ligaments to tear and complete separation of the acromioclavicular joint (Ac).

Trauma may occur from the opposite direction. A fall upon the elbow transmits the stress upward along the shaft of the humerus and rotates the scapula in the opposite direction, causing *elevation* of the acromion at the clavicular end. The ligaments from the coracoid process to the clavicle remain intact, but the acromioclavicular ligaments can tear. The meniscus can also be ruptured by this stress action.

DIAGNOSIS

Degenerative arthritis occurring from trauma to the acromioclavicular joint causes pain over the shoulder region. There is little or no radiation of pain into the arm.[98] Tenderness over the acromioclavicular joint is usual. Movement of the shoulder is pain-free until the scapular phase of the scapulohumeral rhythm involves motion of the scapula. Total elevation of the shoulder girdle such as "shrugging" the shoulder causes pain. Confirmation of the acromioclavicular joint as the source of pain may be made by abolishing the pain with a Novocain injection into the joint. X-rays are difficult to interpret when a frank acromioclavicular separation is not present.

Dislocation of the acromioclavicular joint produces a characteristic deformity known as a "shoulder pointer." The separation permits the scapula to fall away from the clavicle, and the acromion lies below and in front of the clavicle. The outer end of the clavicle can frequently be palpated in the supraspinatus region. If there is merely subluxation of the acromioclavicular joint with injury confined to the acromioclavicular ligaments and the coracoclavicular ligaments remain intact, all

134

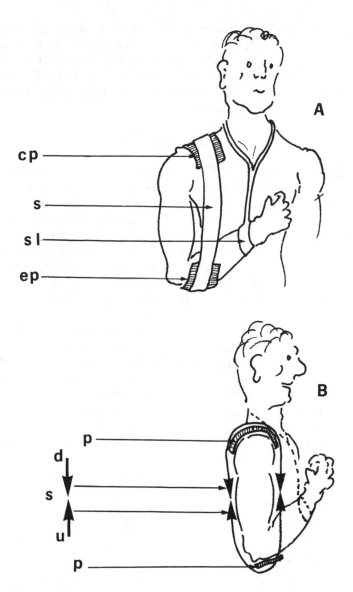

FIGURE 99. Immobilization of acromioclavicular separation: strapping. A. The anterior view in which a circular sling presses down on the clavicle and elevates the arm. A pad protects the clavicle (cp) and the elbow (ep). The wrist is held by a simple sling around the neck (sl). B. The lateral view shows the direction of pull from the circular strap: down upon the clavicle (d), and elevation of the arm (u). If there is no sling, the weight of the arm pulls the acromial fragment down, and the muscles elevate the clavicle, thus separating the acromioclavicular joint. The pads protect the nerves in the shoulder and elbow regions.

that can be seen or palpated is an unduly prominent clavicle. The outer edge of the clavicle "steps" down to the acromion. X-rays suggest subluxation[99] when the acromial and clavicular edges are incongruous in their relationship. X-rays taken of the shoulders with the patient in the upright position, holding weights in both hands, can reveal acromioclavicular separation.

TREATMENT

Simple strapping and comfort slings for 10 days usually suffice in a mild injury. "Simple strapping," however, must be carefully done.[100] The limb is encircled by a strap that elevates the elbow below and depresses the clavicle above. A pad is placed in the axilla. The hand is suspended in a sling from the neck. Pads are placed at the elbow and at the clavicle before strapping to protect against nerve and bony pressure. Immobilization for 3 weeks is indicated if there is subluxation, and 6 weeks if there is complete dislocation (Fig. 99). Reduction and immobilization for the subluxation can be done with a plaster cast.[101]

The treatment of complete dislocation of the clavicle with rupture of the coracoclavicular ligament remains a controversial matter. The present concept favors surgical removal of the distal end of the clavicle and resuture of the ruptured coracoclavicular ligament.[102] This procedure is advocated because most methods of internal fixation of the two opposing articular surfaces (by wire, tendon, or screw) fail to secure a sturdy, pain-free, and moveable joint. The advocates of resection further support their concepts by considering the clavicle to be an "unnecessary" bone.[103]

CHAPTER 8

Biceps Tendinitis and Tear

The kinetics of the biceps was discussed in Chapter 1 and diagrammed in Figure 35. The tendon of the long head of the biceps lies in the bicipital groove of the humerus and at the upper end of the groove angles inward at 90°, thus crossing over the head of the humerus to insert at the upper edge of the glenoid fossa. As shown in Figure 9, it penetrates the cuff in an opening between the supraspinatus tendon and the subscapularis tendons of the cuff. It is invaginated by a downward sleeve of the synovial capsule as it passes under the transverse humeral ligament (see Fig. 5). This ligament holds it within the bicipital groove, and as the tendon passes over the humeral head, it is intra-articular, but extrasynovial.

The relationship of the biceps tendon to the head of the humerus and to the cuff insertion causes it to undergo degenerative changes in association with cuff degeneration. It shares all associated inflammatory dysfunctions of the tissues within the suprahumeral joint.

The biceps tendon does not move within the unmoving humerus. Movement of the tendon is *relative* to the bicipital groove as the groove moves under the tendon (Fig. 35). The greatest displacement of the humerus against the biceps tendon is with the arm internally rotated and elevated in a forward flexed position. In this motion the bicipital groove slides along the tendon toward the insertion on the glenoid; therefore the tendon descends in the groove. When the arm is abducted and flexed backward, the opposite movement occurs, but with a lesser amplitude.

The biceps has no vector force to abduct or elevate the humerus from the dependent position. Only when the arm is externally rotated, which places the biceps muscle and tendon in a straight line, can its muscular action have abducting force. This is a "trick" maneuver learned by patients with paralyzed deltoid muscles and has no effective force.

PATHOLOGY

The tendon of the long head of the biceps undergoes the same attritional changes noted in the cuff tendons. Calcification is rarer in this tendon than in the cuff tendons. Rupture, however, is as common. The direct attachment of the short head of the biceps into the coracoid process makes rupture less frequent. The peculiar angulation and stress points of the long head make rupture here also more frequent than tearing of the insertion upon the bicipital tuberosity of the radius.[104]

The biceps tendon may subluxate or dislocate from the bicipital groove. A cuff tear, capsular tear, and tearing of the transverse bicipital ligament must occur to permit dislocation of the biceps tendon (Fig. 100).

Tenosynovitis of the biceps tendon occurs but is rare and probably occurs with concurrent inflammation of the surrounding cuff structures.

DIAGNOSIS

Pain in the glenohumeral joint region with slight limitation of motion has usually been noted for months or years, indicating degenerative changes in the cuff region. The tendon tears as a painful "snap," followed by swelling and ecchymosis in the region of the bicipital groove below the deltoid muscle. This is followed by the characteristic bulging of the biceps muscle near the antecubital fossa at the lower half of the humerus. There is also a "hollow" where the upper belly of the biceps was. Flexion and supination of the forearm, especially against resistance, increases the bulging at the lower third of the upper arm. Power of forearm supination is decreased, but elbow flexion remains strong because of the remaining short head of the biceps, the brachialis muscle, and the forearm flexors.

If the "snap" is caused by subluxation of the tendon from the bicipital groove rather than tendon tear, there must be an associated capsular tear. In subluxation of the tendon, there is tenderness over the bicipital groove area; the tendon can be snapped by forward flexing and *abducting* the arm, then returning it to the dependent neutral position. Pain radiates down the biceps belly in both avulsion or subluxation of the biceps tendon.

A clinical sign diagnostic of bicipital tendinitis is Yergason's sign,[105] in which pain and tenderness over the bicipital groove is felt when the elbow is flexed and the forearm supinated against resistance or when the elbow is extended, the arm carried backward, and the *forearm*

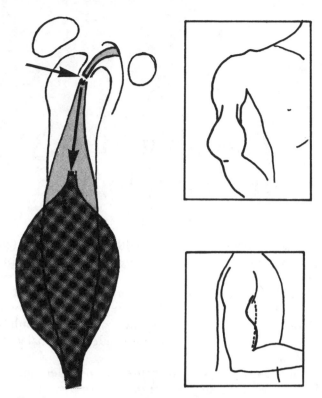

FIGURE 100. Biceps tendon tear. The tendon most frequently tears in its superior portion within the bicipital groove region. The muscle belly bulges in the lower aspect of the humerus. The clinical appearance is shown in the right arm as viewed from the front and the side.

supinated. These signs are of value principally when there is no rupture causing the characteristic "bulging."

TREATMENT

Surgical repair is important only for cosmetic reasons or when forceful supination of the forearm is necessary for the patient's occupation. If repair is indicated, suturing the end of the tendon to the lower portion of the bicipital groove will improve appearance and supination strength. If merely improvement of strength is needed, the end of the tendon can be carried to and attached to the coracoid process.

Disability from a tear of the biceps tendon is usually minimal. After surgical repair, total disability exists for approximately 8 weeks.

CHAPTER 9

The Shoulder
in Hemiplegia

The patient who becomes afflicted with a hemiplegia ("stroke") frequently has involvement of the shoulder that causes disability and frequently causes pain.

Return of function or at least improvement in function of the shoulder is important for resumption of hand function, activities of daily living, safe balance, transfer activities, and effective ambulation. Severe pain in the shoulder may pose a considerable obstacle to successful rehabilitation.

There are numerous factors that influence the adequate return of meaningful function of the upper extremity after a stroke:

1. natural evolutional sequence of recovery;
2. spasticity;
3. development of primitive reflex synergy patterns;
4. apraxia;
5. articular contracture;
6. peripheral sensory deficit;
7. perceptual involvement;
8. intellectual impairment.

Any or all of these factors may be involved in residual impairment and pain.

In patients who suffer hemiplegia the upper extremity usually undergoes various stages in the natural sequence of the involvement. Initially the extremity becomes flail. This may be momentary or persistent with varying decreases of severity or duration.

During the *flail stage* subluxation may occur that adds to the residual disability, contributes to pain, and impairs restoration of function. There are numerous concepts of the causation of subluxation,

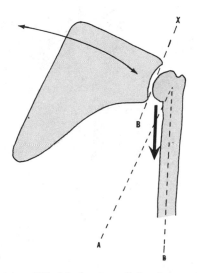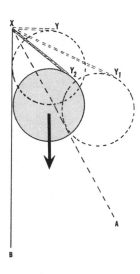

FIGURE 101. Mechanism of glenohumeral subluxation. The diagram at left depicts the change of glenoid angle X–B when the scapula is rotated. The humerus becomes abducted (B) and subluxes downward. The right diagram shows "seating" of the head of the humerus supported by cuff X–Y₁ when the glenoid angle is physiologic X–A. When the scapula rotates, the angle becomes vertical X–B, and the cuff no longer "seats" the head X–Y₂. The humerus subluxes downward.

and attempts at prevention or correction are dependent upon the concept accepted.

The glenohumeral joint maintains its stability by:

1. The angulation of the glenoid fossa, which is dependent upon the position of the scapula on the costal wall.
2. The tone of the supraspinatus muscle within the cuff.
3. The ability of the cuff muscles to contract reflexly upon any abduction of the humerus.
4. The isometric and intermittent isotonic contraction of the deltoid.
5. Possibly the integrity of the superior aspect of the glenohumeral capsule.

If any of the above are impaired, the glenohumeral joint may sublux (Fig. 101).

The change in the angulation of the scapula that alters the normal angle of the glenoid fossa can result from temporary or residual paresis (flaccidity) of the scapular muscles (Fig. 102). Upon cessation of the flaccid stage the onset of spasticity can cause the scapula to rotate downward and forward (Fig. 103).

141

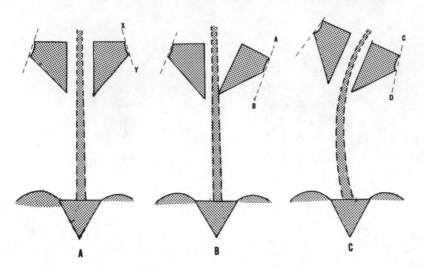

FIGURE 102. Scapular depression. *A*. Scapular alignment with a straight spine (X–Y glenoid angle). *B*. Paresis with downward rotation of the scapula (A–B glenoid angle). *C*. Relative downward rotation of the scapula with functional scoliosis (C–D glenoid angle).

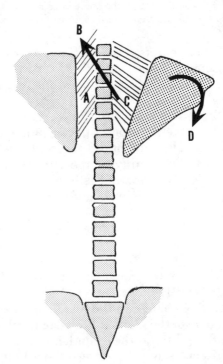

FIGURE 103. Spastic medial scapular muscles. In spasm of the rhomboid muscles that normally rotate the scapula, the glenoid fossa alignment is lowered and the angulation made vertical.

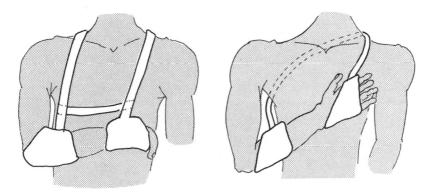

FIGURE 104. Shoulder slings. These slings are designed to support the arm and minimize downward subluxation of the glenohumeral joint. They have not been proven to prevent subluxation and hold the arm in a flexed position.

During the flaccid stage the arm must initially be protected from excessive capsular and cuff stretch caused by the weight of the dependent arm. This is accomplished by means of a sling. The "ideal" sling has yet to be designed or universally accepted. Several types currently used are depicted in Figures 104 through 107.

The corrections required of a splint are:

1. Elevation of the scapula.
2. Seating of the head of the humerus into the glenoid fossa.
3. Elevation support of the humerus.
4. Substitution of the supraspinatus cuff function.

All splints attempt these corrections but fail to do so in part.

The vast majority of "stroke" patients progress into the spastic stage with or without complete development of the flexor synergy (Fig. 108). In this synergy pattern the shoulder remains depressed but assumes an internally rotated, posteriorly flexed position. The remainder of the arm distally has the arm adducted, the elbow flexed, the forearm pronated, and the wrist and fingers flexed. Any or all of these pattern components may be present, but any deviation may occur.

The patient now has resistance to any passive motion and markedly limited active motion in the direction opposed to that of the synergy. Attempting abduction external rotation and elevation of the shoulder may be notably unsuccessful. This attempted motion may also be painful.

Treatment is essentially that of the neurologic sequelae of the "stroke" by one of numerous techniques (e.g., Bobath, P.N.F., Rood).

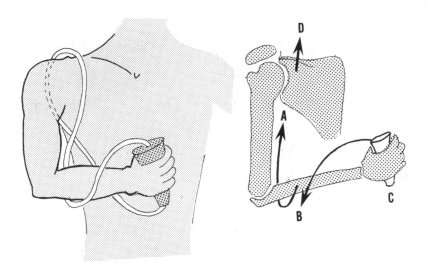

FIGURE 105. Rood sling. The use of elastic tubing gives kinetic support (A) and stimulates extension of the arm. By proper application, the forearm is supinated (B). The hand is held in a cone (C) that spreads the fingers and thumb while radially deviating the wrist. The scapula is elevated and derotated (D).

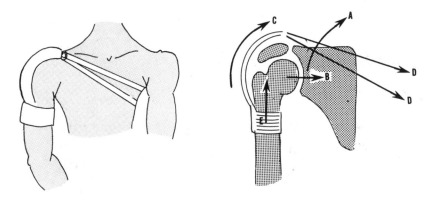

FIGURE 106. Proposed design for prevention of subluxation. A. The glenohumeral joint is elevated to the desired physiologic angulation. B. The head of the humerus is adducted into the "seated" position. C. The humerus is elevated into the suprahumeral fossa. D. The cuff is replaced by the splint. E. The sling attaches to the humerus at the site of deltoid insertion and elevates the humerus into the suprahumeral joint space.

During the flaccid stage techniques to initiate muscular contraction and return of tonus are indicated. If there is sensory deficit the problem is accentuated. Sensory stimulation is attempted by icing, brushing, tapping, rubbing, or even pinching. Any sensory input will conceivably initiate a reflex motor response that ultimately may be

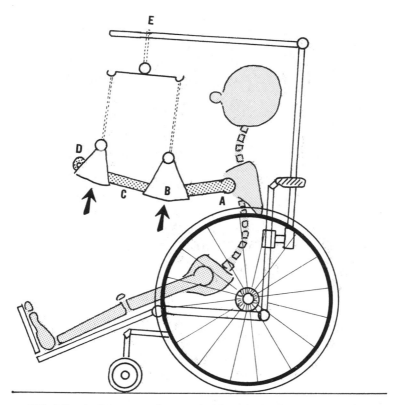

FIGURE 107. Wheel chair arm sling. *A* holds the shoulder forward, flexed, and adducted. *B* supports the elbow in an extended position. *C* and *D* keep the wrist and fingers extended. *E* permits movement of the entire arm.

trained to be under voluntary control. Use of gravity also may initiate motor response. All these techniques must be utilized with full realization that subluxation must be avoided or minimized. They must be used with alternating sling support and with proper positioning when the patient is inactive.

Contracture of the joint(s) is not to be feared during the flaccid stage but may occur with the onset of spasticity. Daily observation and examination of the arm will reveal the onset of spasticity early in the development of the "stroke."

During the phase of flaccidity electrical stimulation of the paretic muscles has value in maintaining muscle fiber integrity as well as being a sensory stimulus. Biofeedback is currently being developed and evaluated in muscle reeducation.

Once spasticity develops the shoulder requires constant positioning. This is to minimize the development of the synergy pattern. The arm must therefore have:

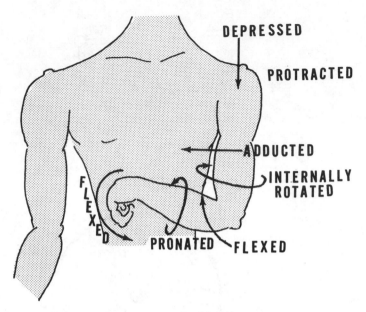

FIGURE 108. Flexor synergy of the upper extremity.

1. The humerus elevated into the glenoid fossa.
2. The shoulder placed in slight abduction, forward flexion, and external rotation.
3. The elbow extended and supinated.
4. The wrist, fingers, and thumb extended, abducted, and supinated.

There are numerous treatment techniques, both in terms of physical and occupational therapy, that have value in treating the spastic stage and initiate neuromuscular reeducation. Specific discussion and evaluation of these numerous techniques are beyond the intent of this text, but some generalizations are warranted.

Of the many modalities ice has proven to give beneficial support in reducing spasticity, especially the prolonged use of ice applied to the spastic muscle.[23] Pattern exercises have been advocated by Knott and Voss,[106] reflex inhibition by Bobath,[107] and numerous other techniques have been promoted, all based upon neurophysiologic concepts.

The predominant pattern that defies amelioration is the persistence of adduction and internal rotation. The opposing patterns of abduction and external rotation of the arm and shoulder not only have weakness as well as inability of initiation, but are restricted by the opposing spasticity of the adductors and internal rotators. Ultimately contracture of the shoulder develops, and passive range of motion is restricted as well as active motion. Pain results.

Hemiplegic pain can be best treated as pain in the shoulder is treated. These pain-relieving procedures include suprahumeral injection of steroids and anesthesia, intra-articular injections of anesthetic agents with or without steroids, suprascapular nerve blocks, and various oral medications. In the spastic shoulder, however, nerve blocks to decrease spasticity have value.

Phenol in diluted solutions, injected into the motor nerves of the spastic muscles or into the motor end plates of the spastic muscles, has many advocates.[108-111]

Depending upon the severity of the spasticity, the use of the tonic neck reflexes is valuable, as is the use of gravity. These have been well documented in the literature.[112]

The shoulder-hand-finger syndrome occurs occasionally in the hemiplegic patient and has characteristics identical to those discussed in Chapter 6.

CHAPTER 10

Visceral Referred Pain

Pain in the region of the shoulder can have its site of origin in a viscus, with the shoulder or scapula as the referred site. To be unaware of this and attribute all pain in the shoulder girdle region to a faulty scapulothoracohumeral mechanism is to miss a potentially serious medical or surgical diagnosis.

Visceral reflex and referred pain to the shoulder region has been widely discussed, although the exact neural mechanism remains speculative. A diseased viscus can refer pain to a remote part of the body: conditions of the diaphragm can cause pain in the neck and shoulder; gallbladder disease can radiate to the shoulder "tip"; gastric disease can refer between the shoulder blades; and angina pectoris or myocardial infarction can be felt in the shoulder, neck, and arm.

A given spinal segment supplies autonomic nerve fibers to a specific viscus, and that same nerve supplies a specific skin area (dermatome). As the viscera become diseased, they set up afferent autonomic impulses *to* the cord that travel (in the cord) to the thalamic center. From the thalamic center the sensation travels to (and is felt in) a somatic (referred) area.[113] These have been described as viscerosensory reflexes. Head[114] mapped out the sensory areas of these cutaneous nerves.

The diaphragm is the most frequent source of extrinsic disease referring pain to the shoulder region. Pain is referred through the phrenic nerve, the afferent fibers of which originate usually in the third and fourth cervical segments (constantly from the C_4 segment and variably from C_3 and C_5).[40] The phrenic nerve has many sites of possible irritation as it descends vertically in front of the anterior scalene muscle through the superior thoracic outlet within the mediastinum, along the pericardium, to finally innervate the superior and inferior surfaces of the central diaphragm. Irritation of the dia-

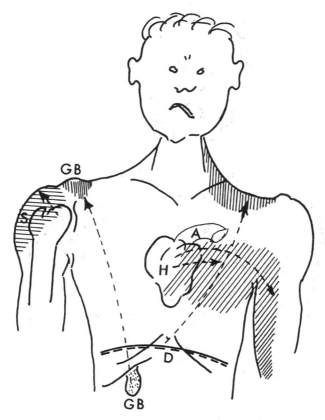

FIGURE 109. Visceral sources of "shoulder" pain. The word "shoulder" is used vaguely in referred pain from visceral sites. Pain that originates in the shoulder is localized directly over the glenohumeral area (S). Irritation of the diaphragm (D) causes referred pain in the trapezius area. Myocardial origin (H and A) refers pain to the axilla and left pectoral region. Gallbladder irritation (GB) refers pain to the tip of the shoulder and posteriorly in the scapular region.

phragm refers pain to the supraclavicular region, the trapezius, and the superior angle of the scapula.[115]

Pulmonary infarction, which involves the diaphragmatic surface of the lung, may cause shoulder pain.[116] Myocardial ischemia via the cardia plexus through the upper four thoracic spinal segments causes referred pain in the infraclavicular and ulnar region. This referred pain is usually left-sided. Involvement of the aortic arch refers to the right side of the neck, whereas the transverse and descending aortic arch refers to the left side of the neck and shoulder.

A perforated abdominal viscus causing pneumoperitoneum will frequently be revealed only by pain in the shoulder area. Gallbladder disease and irritation of the hepatic parenchyma frequently elicit scapular and shoulder pain associated with deep epigastric tenderness. The referred sites of pain from extrinsic sources are diagrammed in Figure 109.

References

1. Codman, E.A.: *The Shoulder.* Thomas Todd, Boston, 1934.
2. DePalma, A.F.: *Surgery of the Shoulder.* ed. 2. J.B. Lippincott, Philadelphia, 1973.
3. Moseley, H.F., and Overgaard, B.: *Anterior capsular mechanism in recurrent anterior dislocation of shoulder: morphological and clinical studies with especial reference to glenoid labrum and glenohumeral ligament.* J. Bone Joint Surg. 44(B):913–927, 1962.
4. Anson, B.J., and McVay, C.B. (eds.): *Surgical Anatomy.* ed. 5. W.B. Saunders, Philadelphia, 1971.
5. Calandriello, B.: *The pathology of recurrent dislocation of the shoulder.* Clin. Orthop. 20:33–39, 1961.
6. Stedman, T.L.: *A Practical Medical Dictionary.* William Wood, Baltimore, 1936.
7. Bloch, J., and Fischer, F.K.: *Acta rheumatologica.* Documenta Geigy (Basel), No. 2, 1961.
8. Moseley, H.F.: *Disorders of the shoulder.* Clin. Symposia 11(3), 1959.
9. Watson-Jones, R.: *Fractures and Joint Injuries, Vol. 11.* ed. 4. Williams & Wilkins, Baltimore, 1960.
10. Kleinberg, S.: *Lesions of the musculotendinous cuff of the shoulder.* J. Bone Joint Surg. 26:50, 1944.
11. Inman, V.E., Saunders, J.B., and Abbott, L.C.: *Observations on the function of the shoulder joint.* J. Bone Joint Surg. 26:1, 1944.
12. Van Linge, B., and Mulder, J.D.: *Function of the supraspinatus muscle and its relation to the supraspinatus syndrome.* J. Bone Joint Surg. 45(B):750–754, 1963.
13. Grant, J.C.: *An Atlas of Anatomy.* ed. 5. Williams & Wilkins, Baltimore, 1962.
14. Hollinshead, W.H.: *Functional Anatomy of the Limbs and Back.* ed. 4. W.B. Saunders, Philadelphia, 1976.
15. DePalma, A.F.: *Degenerative Changes in Sternoclavicular and Acromioclavicular Joints in Various Decades.* Charles C Thomas, Springfield, Ill., 1957.
16. Urist, M.R.: *Complete dislocations of acromioclavicular joint.* J. Bone Joint Surg. 28:813–837, 1946.
17. Decker, J.H.: *Primer on the rheumatic diseases.* J.A.M.A. 190(6):118, 1964.
18. Hirschfeld, A.H., and Behan, R.C.: *Accident process. I. Etiological considerations of industrial injuries.* J.A.M.A. 186:193–199, 1963; *Accident process. II. Toward more rational treatment of industrial injuries.* J.A.M.A. 186:300–306, 1963.
19. McGregor, A.L.: *A Synopsis of Surgical Anatomy.* ed. 6. Williams & Wilkins, Baltimore, 1947.

151

20. Saario, L.: *The range of movement of the shoulder joint at various ages*. Acta Orthop. Scand. 33(4):366–367, 1963.
21. Cailliet, R.: *Low Back Pain Syndrome*. ed. 3. F.A. Davis, Philadelphia, 1981.
22. Moseley, H.F., and Goldie, I.: *The arterial pattern of the rotator cuff of the shoulder*. J. Bone Joint Surg. 45(B), 4, 1963.
23. Hartviksen, K.: *Ice therapy in spasticity*. Acta Neurol. Scand. 38(Suppl. 3): 79–84, 1962.
24. Neviaser, J.S.: *Adhesive capsulitis of shoulder*, in *Instructional Course Lectures of the American Academy of Orthopedic Surgeons*, Vol. 6, 1949, pp. 281–291.
25. Simmonds, F.A.: *Shoulder pain: frozen shoulder*. J. Bone Joint Surg. 31(B): 426, 1949.
26. Patterson, R.L., and Darrach, W.: *Treatment of acute bursitis by needle irrigation*. J. Bone Joint Surg. 19:993, 1937.
27. Shoss, M., and Otto, T.G.: *Roentgen therapy of subdeltoid tendonitis and bursitis: analysis of 159 cases treated with intermediate radiation therapy*. Missouri Med. 52:855–863, 1955.
28. Bonica, J.J.: *The Management of Pain*. Lea & Febiger, Philadelphia, 1954, pp. 310–312.
29. Jampol, H.: *Exercise treatment for the frozen shoulder*. Phys. Ther. Rev. 6:330, 1950.
30. Watson-Jones, R.: *Adhesions of joints and injury*. Br. Med. J., May 1936.
31. Coventry, M.B.: *Problem of painful shoulder*. J.A.M.A. 151(3):177–185, 1953.
32. Steindler, A.: *Lectures on the Interpretation of Pain in Orthopedic Practice*. Charles C Thomas, Springfield, Ill., 1959.
33. Mennell, J.: *The Science and Art of Joint Manipulation, Vol. 1*. J. & A. Churchill, London, 1949.
34. Fisher, A.G.T.: *The frozen shoulder: treatment by manipulation*. Br. J. Phys. Med. 14(3):49–52, 1951.
35. Moseley, H.F.: *Shoulder Lesions*. ed. 3. Churchill Livingstone, Edinburgh, 1969, chap. 9.
36. Quigley, T.B.: *Treatment of checkrein shoulder by use of manipulation and cortisone*. J.A.M.A. 161:850–854, 1956.
37. Quigley, T.B.: *Use of corticosteroids in treatment of painful and stiff shoulder*. Clin. Orthop. 10:182–189, 1957.
38. Cailliet, R.: *Neck and Arm Pain*. ed. 2. F.A. Davis, Philadelphia, 1981, p. 132.
39. Ellis, V.H.: *The diagnosis of shoulder lesions due to injured rotator cuff*. J. Bone Joint Surg. 35(B):1, 1953.
40. Haymaker, W., and Woodhall, B.: *Peripheral Nerve Injuries: Principles of Diagnosis*. ed. 2. W.B. Saunders, Philadelphia, 1953.
41. Kernwein, G.H., Roseberg, B., and Sneed, W.R.: *Arthrographic studies of the shoulder joint*. J. Bone Joint Surg. 39(A):1267–1279, 1957.
42. Samilson, R.L., et al.: *Shoulder arthrography*. J.A.M.A. 175:773–776, 1961.
43. Bateman, J.B.: *The diagnosis and treatment of ruptures of the rotator cuff*. Surg. Clin. North Am. 43(6):1523–1530, 1963.
44. Wolff, H.G., and Wolf, S.: *Pain*. Charles C Thomas, Springfield, Ill., 1951.
45. Mayfield, F.H.: *Causalgia*. Charles C Thomas, Springfield, Ill., 1951.
46. Hanson, E.B.: *Peri-arthritis of the shoulder: studies of vegetative function*. Ann. Rheum. Dis. 11(1):2–16, 1952.
47. Moseley, H.F.: *Shoulder Lesions*. ed. 3 Churchill Livingstone, Edinburgh, 1969, chap. 4.
48. McLaughlin, H.L.: *On the "frozen shoulder."* Bull. Hosp. Joint Dis. 12:383–393, 1951.

49. Neviaser, J.S.: *Adhesive capsulitis of the shoulder: study of pathological findings in periarthritis of the shoulder.* J. Bone Joint Surg. 27:211–222, 1945.
50. McLaughlin, H.L.: *The "frozen shoulder."* Clin. Orthop. 20:126–131, 1961.
51. Enelow, A.J.: *Drug treatment of psychotic patients in general medical practice.* Calif. Med. 102(1):1–4, 1965.
52. Kroegler, R.R.: *Drugs, neurosis, and the family physician.* Calif. Med. 102(1):5–8, 1965.
53. Samilson, R.L.: *Shoulder pain.* Calif. Med. 102(1):23–27, 1965.
54. Simon, W.H.: *Soft tissue disorders of the shoulder.* Orthop. Clin. North Am. 6(2):521, 1975.
55. McGregor, L.: *Rotation at the shoulder: critical inquiry.* Br. J. Surg. 24:425–438, 1937.
56. Quigley, T.B.: *Checkrein shoulder: type of "frozen shoulder." Diagnosis and treatment by manipulation and ACTH or cortisone.* N. Engl. J. Med. 250:188–192, 1954.
57. Frykholm, R.: *Cervical nerve root compression resulting from disc degeneration and root-sleeve fibrosis: a clinical investigation.* Acta Chir. Scand. Suppl. 160.
58. Michele, A.A., and Eisenberg, J.: *Scapulocostal syndrome.* Arch. Phys. Med. Rehabil. 49:383, 1968.
59. Ewad, E.A.: *Interstitial myofibrositis. Hypothesis of the mechanism.* Arch. Phys. Med. Rehabil. 54:449, 1973.
60. Bonica, J.J.: *The Management of Pain.* Lea & Febiger, Philadelphia, 1953, p. 1153.
61. Weinberg, L.M.: *Traumatic myofibrositis: a clinical review of an enigmatic concept.* West. J. Med. 127:99–103, 1977.
62. Kraft, G.H., Johnson, E.W., and LaBan, M.M.: *The fibrositis syndrome.* Arch. Phys. Med. Rehabil. 49:155–162, 1968.
63. Sola, A.E., and Kuitert, J.H.: *Myofascial trigger point pain in the neck and shoulder girdle: 100 cases treated by normal saline.* Northwest Med. 54:980–984, 1955.
64. Cailliet, R.: *Soft Tissue Pain and Disability.* F.A. Davis, Philadelphia, 1977, pp. 142–148.
65. Adson, A.W.: *Cervical ribs: symptoms, differential diagnosis for section of the insertion of the scalene anticus muscle.* J. Int. Coll. Surgeons 16:546, 1951.
66. Lloyd, J.W., and Rosati, L.M.: *Neurovascular compression syndrome of the upper extremity.* Clin. Symposia 10, 1958.
67. Nelson, P.A.: *Treatment of patients with cervico-dorsal outlet syndrome.* J.A.M.A. 127:1575, 1957.
68. Kraus, H.: *Use of surface anesthesia in treatment of painful motion.* J.A.M.A. 116:2582–2583, 1941.
69. Travel, J.: *Ethyl chloride spray for painful muscle spasm.* Arch. Phys. Med. Rehabil. 33:291–298, 1952.
70. Cooper, A.L.: *Trigger point injection: its place in physical medicine.* Arch. Phys. Med. Rehabil. 42:704–709, 1961.
71. Garland, H.C., and Phillips, W. (eds.): *Medicine, Vol. 2.* Macmillan, London, 1953, p. 1461.
72. Poppen, J.L., Kendrich, J.T., and Smith, W.E.: *Cervical rib.* Surg. Clin. North Am. 30:843–851, 1950.
73. Gage, M., and Parnell, H.: *Scalene anticus syndrome.* Am. J. Surg. 73:252–268, 1947.
74. Falconer, M.A., and Weddel, G.: *Costoclavicular compression of the subclavian artery and vein: relation to scalene anticus syndrome.* Lancet 2:539–543, 1943.
75. Kopell, H.P., and Thompson, W.A.: *Pain and the frozen shoulder.* Surg. Gynecol. Obstet. 109:92–96, 1959.

153

76. Kopell, H.P., and Thompson, W.A.: *Peripheral Entrapment Neuropathies.* ed. 2. R.E. Krieger, Huntington, N.Y., 1976.
77. Steinbrocker, O., and Argyros, T.G.: *The shoulder-hand syndrome: present status as a diagnostic and therapeutic entity.* Med. Clin. North Am. 42:1533, 1958.
78. deTakats, G.: *Nature of painful vasodilation in causalgic states.* Arch. Neurol. Psychiatry 50:318, 1943.
79. Kuntz, A., and Farnsworth, D.I.: *Distribution of afferent fibers via sympathetic trunks and gray communicating rami to brachial and lumbosacral plexuses.* J. Comp. Neurol. 53:389–399, 1961.
80. Threadgill, F.D.: *Causalgia.* Bull. Georgetown Univ. Med. Center 11(3):110–112, 1948.
81. Steinbrocker, O., Spitzer, N., and Friedman, N.H.: *The shoulder-hand syndrome in reflex dystrophy of the upper extremity.* Ann. Intern. Med. 29:22–52, 1948.
82. Moberg, E.: *The shoulder-hand-finger syndrome as a whole.* Surg. Clin. North Am. 40(2):367, 1960.
83. Kozin, F., et al.: *The reflex sympathetic dystrophy syndrome.* Am. J. Med. 60:321, 1976.
84. Bonica, J.J.: *The Management of Pain.* Lea & Febiger, Philadelphia, 1953, pp. 420–432.
85. Shaw, R.S.: *Pathological malingering.* N. Engl. J. Med. 271:22–26, 1964.
86. Gellhorn, E., and Loofbourrow, G.N.: *Emotions and Emotional Disorders: A Neurophysiological Study.* Hoeber/Harper, New York, 1963.
87. Bjelle, A., Hagberg, M., and Michaelsson, G.: *Clinical and ergonomic factors in prolonged shoulder pain among industrial workers.* Scand. J. Work Environ. Health 5:205–210, 1979.
88. DePalma, A.F.: *Recurrent dislocation of shoulder joint.* Ann. Surg. 132:1052–1065, 1950.
89. Adams, J.C.: *Review of 180 cases of recurrent dislocation of the shoulder.* J. Bone Joint Surg. 30(B):26, 1948.
90. Moseley, H.F., and Overgaard, B.: *Hermodsson's Roentgenological Studies of Traumatic and Recurrent Anterior and Inferior Dislocations of the Shoulder Joint.* McGill University Press, Montreal, 1963.
91. MacDonald, F.R.: *Intra-articular fractures in recurrent dislocation of the shoulder.* J. Can. Assoc. Radiol. 13, March 1962.
92. Hill, H.A., and Sach, M.D.: *The grooved defect of the humeral head: a frequent unrecognized complication of dislocation of the shoulder joint.* Radiology 35:690–700, 1940.
93. Nash, J.: *Kocher's method of reducing dislocation of the shoulder.* J. Bone Joint Surg. 16:535, 1934.
94. Kirker, J.R.: *Dislocation of shoulder with rupture of axillary vessels.* J. Bone Joint Surg. 34(B):72, 1952.
95. Oppenheimer, A.: *Lesions of the acromioclavicular joint causing pain and disability of the shoulder.* Am. J. Roentgenol. 51:699, 1944.
96. Thorndike, A., and Quigley, T.B.: *Injuries to the acromioclavicular joint.* Am. J. Surg. 55:250, 1942.
97. Poirier, P., and Rieffel, H.: *Mécanisme des luxations subacromiales de la clavicule leur traitement par la suture osseuse.* Arch. Gen. Med. 1:396–422, 1891.
98. Oppenheimer, A.: *Arthritis of the acromioclavicular joint.* J. Bone Joint Surg. 25:807, 1943.
99. King, J.M., Jr., and Holmes, G.W.: *Review of 450 roentgen ray examinations of the shoulder.* Am. J. Roentgenol. 17:214–218, 1927.
100. Jones, R.: *Injuries to joints.* Oxford Medical Publication No. 57, 1924.

101. Urist, M.R.: *Complete dislocation of acromioclavicular joint.* J. Bone Joint Surg. 28:813–837, 1946.
102. Moseley, H.F.: *Athletic injuries to the shoulder region.* Am. J. Surg. 98:401–422, 1959.
103. Gurd, F.B.: *The clavicle is an unnecessary bone. Surplus parts of skeleton: recommendation for excision of certain portions as a means of shortening the period of disability following trauma.* Am. J. Surg. 74:705–720, 1947.
104. Gilcreest, E.L.: *The common syndrome of rupture, dislocation, and elongation of the long head of the biceps brachii.* Surg. Gynecol. Obstet. 38:322, 1934.
105. Yergason, R.M.: *Supination sign.* J. Bone Joint Surg. 13:160, 1931.
106. Knott, M., and Voss, D.: *Proprioceptive Neuromuscular Facilitation: Patterns and Techniques.* ed. 2. Harper & Row, New York, 1968.
107. Bobath, K., and Bobath, B.: *Spastic paralysis: treatment by use of reflex inhibition.* Br. J. Phys. Med. 13(6):121, 1950.
108. Amato, A., Hermsmeyerm C., and Kleinman, K.: *Use of electromyographic feedback to increase inhibitory control of spastic muscles.* Phys. Ther. 53(10):1063, 1973.
109. Mroczek, N., Halpern, D., and McHugh, R.: *Electromyographic retraining in hemiplegia.* Arch. Phys. Med. Rehabil. 59(6):258, 1978.
110. Stockmeyer, S.A.: *An interpretation of the approach of Rood to the treatment of neuromuscular dysfunction.* Am. J. Phys. Med. 46(1):900, 1967.
111. Khalili, A.A., and Betts, H.B.: *Management of Spasticity with Phenol Nerve Blocks.* RD-2529-M. U.S. Department of Health, Education and Welfare, Social Rehabilitation Service, Washington, D.C., 1970.
112. Cailliet, R.: *The Shoulder in Hemiplegia.* F.A. Davis, Philadelphia, 1980.
113. Livingston, W.K.: *Pain Mechanism.* Macmillan, New York, 1943.
114. Head, H.: *On disturbances of sensation with especial reference to the pain of visceral disease.* Brain 16:L-133, 1893.
115. Capps, J.A., and Coleman, G.H.: *Experimental and Clinical Study of Pain in Pleura, Pericardium and Peritoneum.* Macmillan, New York, 1932.
116. Lelan, J.L.: *Visceral aspects of shoulder pain.* Bull. Hosp. Joint Dis. 14:71–73, 1953.

Index

157

158

Shoulder-hand-finger syndrome
  causes of, 108-110
  diagnosis of
    initial manifestations in, 113-115
    stages in, 117-119
    sympathetic nervous system in-
      volvement in, 115-116
  evolution of, 111, 115
  pathophysiology of, 110-113
  psychiatric aspects of, 122-124
  reflex sympathetic dystrophy and,
    109, 115-117
  treatment of
    physical therapeutic techniques
      in, 121-122
    stellate ganglion block in, 120-
      121
Shoulder joint. See Glenohumeral
    joint.
Slings, types of, 143, 144, 145
Spasticity, hemiplegic, treatment of,
    145-147
Spinal cord tumor, 93-94
Stellate ganglion nerve block, 120-
    121
Sternoclavicular joint, 2, 31-32
"Stiff shoulder." See "Frozen shoul-
    der."
"Stroke," shoulder function and. See
    Hemiplegia, shoulder func-
    tion and.
Subluxation
  hemiplegia and, 140-141
  sling to prevent, 144
Subscapularis muscle, 12-13
Superior pulmonary sulcus tumors,
    105
Suprahumeral joint, 2-3
  components of, 10
  nature of, 9
Suprascapular nerve block, 57, 64-65
Suprascapular nerve entrapment, 106
Supraspinatus muscle, 11-12
  function of, 19-20
Sympathetic referred pain
  causes of, 108-110
  diagnostic considerations in, 113-
    119

management of, 119-122
pathophysiologic mechanisms of,
    110-113
psychiatric aspects of, 122-124
upper extremity circulation and,
    108-109
Synergy, flexor, 143, 146
Synovial capsule, glenohumeral, 6-9

TENDINITIS
  abduction and, 39, 42
  aging and, 42
  bicipital, 137-139
  calcific, 43-45
  causes of, 38-39
  diagnosis of, 48-53
  treatment of. See Musculoskeletal
    pain, treatment of.
Teres minor muscle, 12
Transverse humeral ligament, 13-14
Trapezius muscle
  lower, 23
  upper, 22
Traumatic pain. See Acromioclavicu-
    lar joint, lesions of; Disloca-
    tion.
"Trigger points"
  pain diagnosis and, 50
  postural fatigue and, 97, 98, 99
Tumors
  pulmonary sulcus, 105
  spinal cord, 93-94

VISCERAL referred pain
  abdominal perforated viscus and,
    149
  diaphragm and, 148-149
  gallbladder disease and, 149-150
  gastric disease and, 148
  hepatic parenchymal irritation and,
    149-150
  pulmonary infarction and, 149
  sources of, diagram of, 149

WEITBRECHT, foramen of, 8-9
Wheel chair arm sling, 145

YERGASON'S sign, 138-139